Rudy & Connie,

I pray that this book
brings much health &
happiness for both of you.

Thank you for being such
wonderful parents
over the years!

God Bless

1-12-10

NINE
SECRETS
—OF—
HEALTH

Unlocking All Your God Given Power to Heal

S. DON KIM

Book Cover Design by Dan Yeager   www.nu-images.com
Interior Design by Casey Hooper   www.caseyhooperdesign.com
Illustrations by Kevin McCarthy   www.kmcreative.net
Contribution by Emily Hohenwarter
Edited by Karla Bergstrom

LCCN: 2009909819
ISBN-13 978-0-9819628-0-1

Printed in the United States of America

This book is dedicated to . . .

The Almighty Father, God, who gave
me a new life, a new passion, and
a new purpose seven years ago.

My lovely wife, Robin, whose actions allow me to
experience God's love firsthand,
and who makes everything I do possible.
She is my best friend, my life partner,
my advisor, and my love.

My mother, Yun, and father, Byung, who taught
me to be right no matter what.

My sisters, Sue and Jackie, who
have always been there for me.

CONTENTS

Nine Secrets of Health
INTRODUCTION

Thank you for taking the time to pick up this book. Your action shows that you care enough about yourself to get healthy. You've already made a giant step toward a healthy life in flipping to this page. I commend you.

Now that you've made the first step, it's time to read through and apply my principles for the **ultimate life makeover**. Once you've finished this book, I hope you have a good idea of what my nine secrets entail. But if you want to learn more, don't worry. There will be many more books to follow this one, and each will explain a secret in further detail.

For now, however, let's focus on the pages in your hands. I hope this book educates, inspires, and enlightens everyone who reads it to make changes. I hope you make changes in the way you **eat** and **drink**. I hope you make changes in the way you **move**. I hope you make changes in the way you **think**. I hope you make changes in the way you **feel**. And, most of all, I hope you make changes in the way you **believe**. A new outlook in all of these components is required for health, and I hope to be the one who can help you change your perspective. **You have the power to change your health.** I am going to show you how. Are you ready?

WHY AM I TALKING ABOUT HEALTH?

"You are a foot doctor; why are you talking about health? Why don't you just stick to feet?" People ask me that all the time. Well, I was sticking to feet earlier in my medical career. During the first five years of my practice, that was exactly what I was doing. I became very busy, seeing patients and doing lots of foot surgeries as my practice grew. As I was performing more and more surgeries, I had to deal with many more complications in my patients too.

One day, I was totally hit by depression. When I saw the patient schedule on that day, I saw so many names of patients who were still limping around with crutches, boots or wooden shoes after they'd undergone my surgeries. Many of them had had operations months ago! No matter what I did, they were not getting better. They had thick scars, bones that did not heal, and joints that would not move. They were what we called "practice builders." They kept coming and paying bills, but seeing them made me feel horrible about my surgical skills.

"I am an awful foot doctor! I need to quit," I thought. I was convinced that I should resign. I became fearful of doing surgeries and kept thinking about possible complications that would result. Were these people's problems my fault? One night after a long day of seeing patients, I decided to find out what I did wrong. I pulled out about 50 patient charts and spread them on my desk. Since the patients had been coming for a while, their charts were so thick they covered my entire desk. I was literally buried under a mass of charts.

I started to look through all the charts one by one. After several hours, I yelled, "Hallelujah! It is not my fault after all." I was overjoyed. I realized that I was looking through the charts of sick patients. When I did surgeries on **diabetic, hypertensive, obese, arthritic,** and **multiply medicated patients,** they never got better. It took so long for them to recover, if they ever recovered at all. Of course, there were cases when I made mistakes or did not do the surgeries properly. However, the majority of complications from these cases were not my fault.

"How do I get my patients healthier so they can have minimal complications from my surgeries?" I thought. I remember it was the summer of 1995 when I started to search for this answer. It has been my obsession since that time. I read every book I can get my hands on about healing. I looked at Chinese medicine that uses herbs and needles and has been around for the last 5000 years. I read about Ayurvedic medicine from India, where they treat every disease with food. They have 8,000 years of healing history. Doing just what Hippocrates said 2500 years ago, "**Use food as medicine,**" they heal every ailment. I studied nutrition, exercise physiology, emotional healing, and spiritual healing. One day I screamed again, "Hallelujah!"

GOD GAVE YOU ALL THE POWER TO HEAL YOURSELF

Here's what I found out since that evening of depression in my office: **we are designed to heal ourselves from any disease!** We can heal ourselves of all our medical problems, from the common cold to cancer and everything in between. It is truly a miracle!

I was trained in allopathic medicine, and according to that discipline, there are 40,000 known diseases and 58,000 different medications with which to treat them.[1] I was trained to use surgery and medication to treat illnesses. And I still believe that these things are necessary to treat some problems. However, when you depend on drugs and surgery as the only means of healing, you will have no power to heal yourself. You will get weaker and sicker. You have to believe in your own power to heal and not put your faith in outside sources. Only then will you be transformed.

I found out that we are designed by God, the master designer, to be perfectly healthy without any medications. But only if we do nine things right. These things are the nine secrets of health; the title of this book. When you hear the nine secrets, you will probably think that they aren't really "secret." Really, they're common sense. Still, the nine things are not practiced by many people, and that is why I call them secrets. When you understand the nine secrets, you will realize that you are so powerful just as you are, the way God designed and created you. You will not be afraid of diseases anymore, as you will know what to do with your body, mind, and spirit to overcome any sickness.

The purpose of this book is to **empower you to take control of your health.** I have seen many miracles happen through my seminars when my patients began practicing the nine secrets in their lives. Unlock the healing power that you already have by reading these pages ahead and embracing these secrets.

YOU ARE SO AMAZING

Have you ever stopped to think about how complex and perfect your body is? It's absolutely phenomenal. Your heart beats more than 100,000 times each day; that's about 3 billion beats over an average lifetime![2] With each pump, it sends about 1/3 cup of blood through your body, delivering oxygen along more than 60,000 miles of veins, arteries, and capillaries, which is twice the distance around the world.[3] [4]

Now, think about your eyes. They're a miracle! Amazingly, through the work of millions of cells, your eyes are able to see. And not only can you see, but you can also discern depth and color. In fact, you have 120 million rod cells that are solely dedicated to giving you night vision.[5] Miraculous functions happen all over your body. Think about your nose, taste buds, muscles, and skin: they are all complex. Each of your many parts works perfectly to keep you alive. You are a complicated-yet-perfect work of art!

Now reflect on how much you've changed over your lifetime. You started out as a tiny two-celled zygote, a fertilized egg, and now you are a full-grown human being! Now, you have more than 75 trillion cells in your body, and each one is alive and has a specific job.[6] Some cells make up muscles; they help keep you strong and active. Other cells make up your skin, which protects you from the elements. Your skin is constantly regenerating, with billions of new cells being made every day to keep you healthy.[7] Your body is also stocked with trillions of red blood cells. In fact, about 200 billion (200,000,000,000) red blood cells are produced in your body every day, which equates to 2.4 million (2,400,000) red blood cells a second![8] These special cells carry oxygen all over your body. Although they are microscopic, they are a big reason you are alive.

It's amazing to think about how we work! And it's even more amazing to think how you are constantly renewing yourself. Your cells are reborn daily. In fact, your stomach lining completely regenerates every three to five days.[9] Your skin is all new every 28 days.[10] Even our bones are regularly made new; in fact, we replace our entire skeletons about every seven years![11]

Since your cells are constantly changing, **you have the power to change your health**. A new cell has great potential. Don't let your new cells be stricken with toxins and disease. Change your lifestyle to change your cells and change your health.

WHEN YOUR CELLS ARE HEALTHY, YOU ARE HEALTHY.

In your body, there are approximately one trillion cells per every one kilogram of body weight.[12] That means if you weigh 132.2 pounds (60 kilograms), you have 60 trillion cells! Believe it or not, when you were conceived, you were just 2 cells: one from your mom and one from your dad. After nine months in your mother's womb, you grew to around 3.6 trillion cells. You made 274 different types of cells from your first two stem cells.[13] When all 274 different kinds of cells—skin cells, bone cells, brain cells, and many more—communicate and work in harmony, you are healthy. Now, **you are a community of trillions of cells** that live and thrive. On the other hand, if your cells are not healthy and working in harmony—you become sick.

Let's look at an example of one of your cells. In the illustration, you can see a few basic parts of your cell anatomy. All of your cells have a nucleus, which contains your DNA. Your DNA contains the codes for your genes. DNA is also the template used to create RNA, which, in turn, is used to make proteins. But it gets more complicated than this basic relationship. I will go into more detail about how DNA works in a few sections below. You can also see mitochondria in the drawing of the cell. Mitochondria are your energy centers; they are where ATP is produced. ATP powers many reactions in your body,

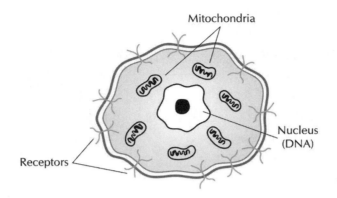

and it is commonly known as the "energy currency" of your cells. That is, whenever your cells need to do something, they must "spend" a little ATP to make it happen.

Finally, in the picture you can see the receptors that are embedded in the cell membrane. These receptors look a bit like antennae, and they're very important. For the longest time, scientists thought the nucleus was the brain that controlled the functions of the cells. Recently, however, they realized that it is the membrane and its receptors that act like the brain of all cells. DNA is just the reproductive system that produces new cells, not the brain—it doesn't control most day-to-day functions.[14]

IT IS NOT YOUR GENES!

In 2003, the **Human Genome Project** was completed. It took 13 years, 3,000 scientists from all over the world, and an exorbitant $3 billion to finish. In the project, the scientists mapped out 3 billion sequences of human DNA.[15] They wanted to find the exact sequence of all our genes. This was quite an undertaking!

As you can see in the illustration, your DNA is tightly wound into X-shaped structures called chromosomes. There are millions of base pairs on each chromosome. With 46 total chromosomes grouped in 23 pairs, humans have billions of total base pairs in their genetic code. Scientists expected to find hundreds of thousands of genes in our DNA. Genes code for proteins, and since we have 100,000 different proteins in each of our cells and 20,000 regulatory proteins that turn on or off each gene, they expected to see at least 120,000 genes total. Shockingly, they only found 23,688 genes.[16]

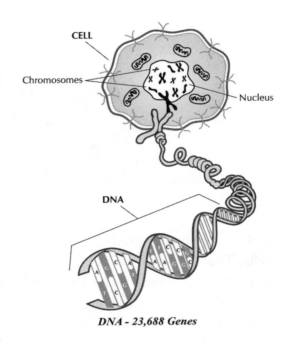

DNA - 23,688 Genes

It turns out that we have fewer genes than a round worm, an organism that has only 969 total cells. Round worms have 24,000 genes; fruit flies have 15,000 genes.[17] Previously, scientists theorized that every function of the human body was controlled by its own gene. They were dumbfounded when they discovered that this couldn't be true.[18]

THE NEW SCIENCE OF EPIGENETICS

Since the time of the Human Genome Project, we have learned that your 23,688 genes can make more than 100,000 different types of proteins in each of your cells. What does this mean? It means that your genes do not determine what proteins to produce; something above and beyond your genes is responsible for this decision. This is called "**epigenetics.**" "Epi" means above, and, therefore, epigentics means above the control of the genes. Because of epigenetics, your health is controlled by the environment that your cells are in. This is one of the hottest topics in natural medicine today.[19]

With so much new information coming onto the scene, everything about genetic science has changed. Until recently, the same dogma about DNA had been upheld since its structure was discovered in 1953. This dogma stated that DNA's job was to code for RNA, which codes for protein. That basic relationship was very straightforward. However, with the discovery of epigenetics, the situation gets a bit more complicated. Now, scientists don't think protein production necessarily begins with DNA. Instead, **environmental signals** start the process of creating protein. But the system is all interlinked, as you can see in the illustration. An environmental signal will release a regulatory protein, which will turn a gene off or on. When the gene is turned on, the DNA will be used to create RNA, which will be used to make a new protein. In the new model, the code for every protein is still held within DNA. Even regulatory proteins are produced by DNA. It's just

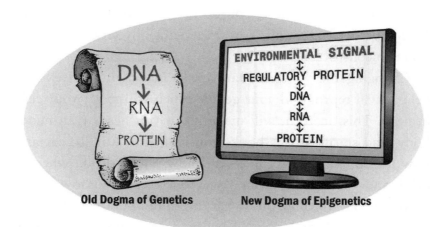

Environmental Control over DNA

that the environment plays the biggest role in determining which proteins get produced at any given time.

Each gene can create 2,000 or more variations of protein from the same genetic blueprint.[20] Only 5 percent of the proteins your cells make are controlled by genetics. The other 95 percent of proteins are turned on and off by the environment.[21] **Your body's inner emotional, mental, energetic, biochemical and spiritual environments are what activate and express your genes.** Outer influences like your interaction with other people, the food you eat, and the toxins you come into contact with also determine which genes will be turned on to be expressed.[22] The bottom line: it's not your genes that are controlling you; it's your own decisions.

YOUR LIFESTYLE DETERMINES YOUR HEALTH

Your inner and outer environments together make up your lifestyle. When you change your lifestyle for the better, your healthy genes will be turned on to express a healthy body, mind, and spirit. This is what this book is all about. Unlike what you have thought in the past, you do not have to be a **victim** of genetic predetermination. You are a **victor** of your own destiny. You can control your health!

Changing the way you eat, drink, move, think, feel, and believe will reprogram your genes, which will make your cells healthy. This, in turn, will make all of you healthy, in mind, body, and spirit. In this book, you will learn how to eat and how not to eat; how to drink and how not to drink; when to drink and when not to drink; how to exercise and how not to exercise; what to think and what not to think; how to feel and how not to feel; and what to believe and how not to believe. With these tips, you will be in control of your health!

HOW TO GET THE MOST
OUT OF THIS BOOK

Before you begin reading about the secrets to health, you need to understand the following foundational principles, which are included in every chapter of this book. These are the take-away lessons from my secrets, and if you follow these basic guidelines, you'll be doing everything you need to do for a healthy life.

1. NATURAL IS GOOD, PROCESSED IS NOT. Throughout this book, I'll be encouraging you to eat natural foods and to do things the natural way. "Natural" means things that haven't been altered by man. **In other words, if God made it, eat it. If men made it, don't eat it.** Recognizing that all kinds of processing—in foods, water, cooking, and light is bad—will make a huge difference in your health.

2. BE PROACTIVE TO BE HEALTHY. Don't wait until problems arise to make a change. By then, you will already be suffering. Make positive changes now! Drink before you get thirsty. Eat before you get hungry. Move before you get stiff. Laugh before you get depressed. Believe before you get fearful.

3. ELIMINATE TOXINS TO IMPROVE HEALING POWER. Toxins diminish healing power. Eliminating toxins will help you create the environment necessary to change your health. Cut out toxic foods, drinks, thoughts, feelings, beliefs, and people from your life.

4. INCREASE YOUR METABOLISM TO STAY FIT AND SLIM. When your metabolism works at a fast rate, you burn energy more efficiently and lose weight. Use water, greens, supplements, exercise, restful sleep, laughter, and forgiveness to crank the engine of your metabolism to an all time high.

5. KEEP YOUR BLOOD STREAM CLEAN TO LOOK YOUNGER AND HEALTHIER. Your blood is what keeps you alive. Make sure your **river of life** is clean so nutrients can be supplied where they are needed and toxins can be readily released from your body. Supply more water, greens and supplements to your blood stream to give it cleaning power. Eliminate processed sugar and processed fats to make sure your blood doesn't get filled with grime in the first place.

6. SCHEDULE AND SCORE. At the end of each chapter, you'll see charts that will ask you to **schedule your health** and **score your wellness**. These activities are a fun way to see how you measure up to ideal health practices. If you meet the wellness threshold described in the activities, you'll get one point. There are 10 total points available in this book. Use the chart below to help determine your oveall health:

POINTS	RESULTS
9-10	Consider yourself healthy!
6-8	You'd be healthier if you made serious changes
5 or less	You need a complete lifestyle overhaul

7. NINE WEEK PROGRAM. Another way to take advantage of all this book has to offer is to follow a timeline. After you've read the book once looking for the above principles, you can go through it a second time over **nine weeks**, as the program was designed to do. Ideally, every secret will take a week to master before you can move on to the next secret. The best way to go through the nine-week program is to get a **partner** and commit to following the nine secrets together. Remember to tell your family and

close friends that you will be going through this program and **solicit emotional encouragement and support.** Also, get a notebook or a journal to record your actions and feelings along the way. In my experience, people who keep journals usually stick through the program and finish with a new outlook on life.

8. CELEBRATE EVERY WIN you have over the course of the program, even the little ones that aren't noticeable to other people. For example, a small victory would be successfully eliminating soda from your diet. You might also want to set weight-loss goals and commend yourself each time you meet one.

9. PARTICIPATE IN THE SEMINAR. If you feel you need a more **organized way** to go through the program, go to **www.9WeekTransformation.com,** where you will find dates of upcoming programs led by me or other facilitators. In these seminar-based experiences, you will be assigned a partner if you don't have one already. You'll also be given an experienced leader who will coach you and help you through the program.

10. CLEAN UP DAY. One last thing: set a date to get the nine-week program started. In addition, set another date for an **OUT with the OLD and IN with the NEW day.** This is the day to clean out your refrigerator, pantry, and cupboards and stock your home with more live foods. Have fun!

Chapter 1

OUR UNIVERSE,
YOUR UNIVERSE

From the smallest invisible particles of quantum and atoms to the largest planetary systems of galaxies, all things in the universe are made in mirror images of one another. They are all made of nine elements of body, mind and spirit. When you embrace the invisible energy of spirit that controls every level of the universe, you will be able to attain perfect health.

THE FRACTAL GEOMETRY OF NATURE

Fractal geometry is a revolutionary breakthrough in the way we view the reality of nature.[23] It all began in 1975, when an IBM computer scientist named Dr. Benoit Mandelbrot discovered a geometric pattern in his work. Mandelbrot dubbed this new geometric pattern "fractal geometry." The term was derived from the Latin "fractus," which means broken, fragmented, and discontinued.[24] Unlike the standard **Euclidean geometry,** which

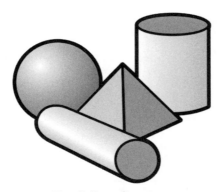

Euclidian Geometry

showed nature as being round and symmetrical, fractal geometry proved that nature is truly composed of uneven shapes. It also showed that every feature of an image is connected, shrunk or expanded by exactly the same ratio.[25] In other words, all things are made up of smaller parts, which look exactly like the larger whole.

The discovery of fractal geometry coincides with the cosmologic principle formalized by Einstein and E. A. Milne, which states that the laws of nature must everywhere and always be the same.[26] Basically, Mendelbrot found the hidden order underlying the shapes of everything in nature.[27] This is truly what it means to be **"as above, so below"** and **"as within, so without."**

Let's look at an example of this phenomenon in nature.

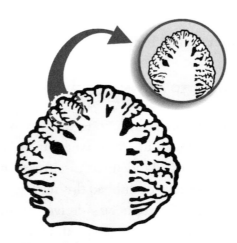

Fractal Geometry in Cauliflower

Think about **cauliflower**, which is shown in the picture to the left. When you cut cauliflower in half, you will notice that every small branch looks identical to the whole cauliflower.[28] And within each small branch, there are even more little offshoots that match the primary shape. All the parts are connected, with the smallest branches seeming to be imitations of the plant as a whole.

THE FRACTAL NATURE OF YOUR BODY

Your body is built the same way as that cauliflower, although it is much more complex. For example, your **lungs** maximize their surface area through fractal geometry. The area where oxygen is exchanged in your lungs, called the alveoli, is the size of a tennis court. However, it is crammed into a space with a volume equivalent to just a few tennis balls.[29] How do our lungs manage to fit in such a small space? They do it by curving around through an almost infinite fractal structure. You can see a picture of this in the illustration below. Similarly, your arteries, which make up just 3 percent of the body's volume, can reach every cell in your body because of fractal geometry.[30]

Chinese medicine has recognized the principles of fractal geometry for thousands of years. The ancient Chinese knew that your ears, hands, and feet are made in an identical way to the

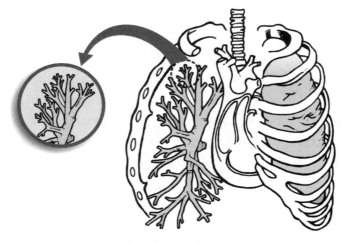

Fractal Nature of Lungs

rest of your body. In fact, my father-in-law, who is an amazing acupuncturist, uses needles only on the hands to treat ailments all over the body. I myself use feet to figure out the functions and structures of the whole body. I will talk more about this in the exercise chapter later in this book, when I explain the relationship between your feet and your spine.

SIX KNOWN LEVELS OF THE UNIVERSE

In my observations, I have realized that there are six known levels to the universe. All of these levels are composed of similar structures, just like in fractal geometry. The smaller levels are identical in composition to the larger levels, and in each level, there are three overriding elements that can be considered equivalent to body, mind and spirit. On the levels that are most familiar to us, our bodies have the illusion of being most important. But as we can see from higher and lower levels, this isn't true. The spirit is infinitely more powerful.

You can see a visual of the six levels in the illustration on page 7. I'll explain each of them, starting all the way in outer space and ending in the deepest part of who you are.

1. GALAXIES. There are at least 250 billion suns within our galaxy alone, and there are trillions of galaxies within the observed universe.[31] There are stars, clusters of stars, galaxies, clusters of galaxies, and super clusters of galaxies in outer space.[32] Each galaxy has a core, with millions of stars that rotate around it. Each star has its own satellite as well. The core is the spirit—it controls the entire galaxy universe.

2. SOLAR SYSTEM. In our solar system, the **sun** is at the center and planets rotate around it. Our earth is the third rock from

the sun, and it has a moon rotating around it. The **earth** represents the physical aspect of our solar system; it is similar to our bodies. The **moon** is like our head, which contains the mental aspects of thinking and feeling. The sun is the spirit that controls the entire solar universe. It is 1.3 million times bigger than the earth, and with its invisible energy, it controls the rotation and the course of the earth's travel.

3. HUMAN BODY. This is the universe that we are most familiar with. Your **body** is made up of 60 to 100 trillion cells, which work in perfect synchronicity as a community. Your **mind** has conscious thoughts and an emotional subconscious, which controls most of your life. Behind the physical and mental parts of us, the superconscious exists. This is the spiritual aspect of who we are, and it controls the universe of our bodies. You might not realize that you have a superconscious mind that guides you. However, this superconscious is infinitely powerful. It is your **spirit,** and it will help you know God.

4. CELLS. Your cells have **receptor proteins** in their membranes, or coverings. These receptors are the brains of the cells; they receive environmental information. Your cells' receptor proteins are equivalent to your thoughts and emotions. Your cells' **cytoplasm** is like the body of the cells; it has **mitochondria,** which are the energy factories of the cells, just like the heart is the energy center of the body. The **effector proteins** and the **DNA** of the cells carry out the built-in programs of DNA replication and protein production under the control of the spirit. It is this innate program of the spirit that controls which genes become turned on or off. If healthy information is provided, healthy genes get turned on to produce healthy cells. If unhealthy environmental information is given, unhealthy

cells result. Your cellular universe is controlled by this invisible program of spiritual energy.

5. ATOMS. "Atom" means invisible in Greek.[33] Atoms are mostly empty space, with a nucleus occupying about one billionth of their total volume.[34] Think of all that empty space as the atom's spirit. It makes up most of the "structure," but we don't even recognize it as anything more than emptiness. However, atoms are made out of invisible energy, not tangible matter.[35] And that invisible energy is the spirit that controls this atomic universe.

6. QUANTUM. According to Einstein, matter is made up of mostly energy. We know that energy fields are influential in controlling our physiology and our health.[36] There is empty space, which is composed of energy, between all particles in the universe. This empty space is known as quantum.[37] It's like a tornado: with a tornado, you only see the particles that are flying around within it, not the energy of the tornado itself. This energy that you don't see is quantum. The quantum world exists within and behind the solid world that we can see and touch, beyond our normal spectrum of perception.[38] This is the spiritual world that controls your purely energetic quantum universe.

YOU ARE A MIRROR IMAGE
OF THE WHOLE UNIVERSE

In this book, we will mainly explore three of the six known levels of the universe, namely our solar system; your body, mind, and spirit; and your cells. All three of these levels of the universe are interconnected and are mirror images of one another, so in talking about one we are really talking about all. My nine secrets speak in terms of the solar system, but they are meant to

Six Known Levels of Universe

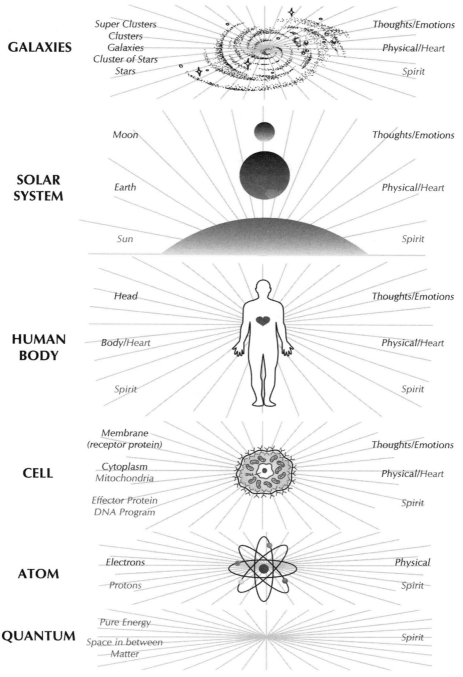

GALAXIES

Super Clusters
Clusters
Galaxies
Cluster of Stars
Stars

Thoughts/Emotions

Physical/Heart

Spirit

SOLAR SYSTEM

Moon

Earth

Sun

Thoughts/Emotions

Physical/Heart

Spirit

HUMAN BODY

Head

Body/Heart

Spirit

Thoughts/Emotions

Physical/Heart

Spirit

CELL

Membrane
(receptor protein)

Cytoplasm
Mitochondria

Effector Protein
DNA Program

Thoughts/Emotions

Physical/Heart

Spirit

ATOM

Electrons

Protons

Physical

Spirit

QUANTUM

Pure Energy
Space in between
Matter

Spirit

be applied to all levels of your life. Five of my secrets deal with your body, which is equivalent to the earth in the solar system. There are five elements to the earth, just like there are five elements to our bodies. The next secret, wind, talks about how to use your body in exercise. The remaining three secrets pertain to your mind and spirit.

WHAT ARE THE NINE ELEMENTS THAT MAKE UP THE NINE SECRETS?

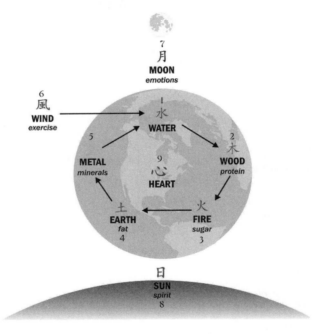

9 Elements of the Solar System

The first element, water, is the simplest of all. You need to "super hydrate" to maximize your health. **Water** is the most abundant element on earth, and it makes up most of your body. To avoid the problems associated with unclean water, you've got to drink a lot and drink often.

Wood is the second element of the earth, and in your body, it refers to the protein you eat, particularly from greens. The secret here is to eat the greenest green vegetables and to make sure you get plenty of protein and phytonutrients in your diet. Many people think that protein has to come from animal products like meat and dairy. But in reality, green vegetables provide the building blocks you need to make all the protein your body requires.

The third element of the earth, **fire**, corresponds with sugar. The earth needs a good amount of fire in its core to keep going, but too much fire and the whole world could be destroyed. Similarly, you need sugar for energy, but when you eat too much sugar, your body is on fire and in danger. For health, you need to reduce the amount of processed sugar you consume, relying instead on natural carbohydrates.

Earth, the fourth element, relates to fat. Just as our planet is covered with a crust of earth, so are you covered with fat. It makes up your hair, fingernails, and organ membranes. You need fat to stay alive, but too much of it can lead to health problems. Increasing the natural fat you eat will make you healthier.

Finally, the fifth element of earth is **metal**, and it relates to the health secret of vitamins and minerals. Supplementing your diet with daily vitamins and minerals will help nourish your body. The earth is filled with a multitude of naturally occurring vitamins and minerals, and you need to fill your body with them too.

These five dietary elements make up a healthy body, just like the five elements of earth make up a balanced system. But as with the earth, factors external to the body make a difference too. Think about **wind** and how it's related to the earth. It's not a part of the earth, but it's intimately connected. Wind comes from movement. In the nine-element human system, then, wind is equivalent to exercise. So that's the sixth element—get moving!

The remaining three secrets correspond to other elements in the solar system. The **moon** is number seven, and it stands for our thoughts and emotions. Like the moon, which pulls the waters of the earth through tides, our thoughts and emotions have a great effect on our bodies. We can't ignore them. But learning to understand our thoughts and emotions and control their influence is crucial for a healthy life. The moon doesn't produce light; it only reflects the light of the sun. Similarly,

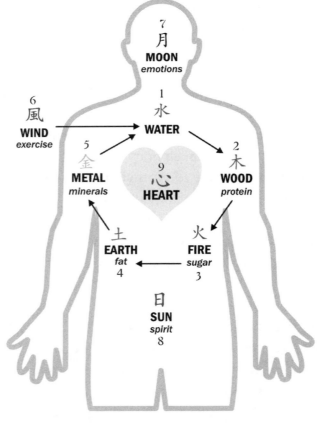

9 Elements of the Body

we have to realize that our thoughts and emotions are not the source of happiness. True happiness comes from divine love.

God's **love** is the eighth element of health, and it's equivalent to the sun. The **sun** is what allows life to exist on earth; similarly, God's love is what makes human life possible. Whether we accept it or not, God's love for us is unconditional. It is the source of all. It is the **spirit**.

This brings me to the ninth element of health, which is the most crucial and also the most difficult to grasp—**belief**, or, as I will refer to it in this book, **heart**. We have to believe in God's love whole heartedly for optimal health. We have to allow Him to show us our purpose in life. If we follow the other secrets to health, we'll improve our well being, but without believing in God's love, we will never realize our full potential. Believing in God will allow Him to cure all of our problems. We will have a perfect environment, one which is conducive to changing our genes to our advantage.

Throughout this book, you will learn all about my nine secrets and how they can change your body, mind, and spirit. Most importantly, you will learn that the quantum level of the universe exists within your own universe of atoms and cells and within our outer universe of galaxies. It is the invisible force created by energy fields that is in control of the whole universe. This is called the energy of God. More accurately, it is the loving energy of God. Once you embrace this **universal energy of God** into your heart, you will be able to attain perfect health in your mind, body, and spirit.

Chapter 2
THE 1ST SECRET:
WATER

"SUPER-HYDRATE, SHOWER FROM WITHIN"

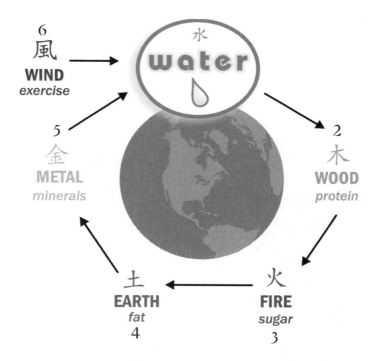

70 percent of our earth is covered with water. Our bodies are also 70 percent water. Water is essential for the creation of life. Dehydration is by far the most devastating health risk for everyone. When you are well hydrated, your metabolism works better, your body is detoxified, and you are safe from most diseases.

However, when water is processed through different methods, it is devitalized of its powerful healing properties. Let's super hydrate to keep our bodies clean and healthy!

DID YOU TAKE A SHOWER TODAY?

You wouldn't go a day without cleaning the outside of your body, so why do so many of us **neglect to clean our insides?** We build up gunk in our insides just from day-to-day use, similar to how our hair or skin gets dirty. We have to shower on the inside like we shower on the outside. And just how can we shower from within? By drinking water. Drink water to clean your body, inside and out.

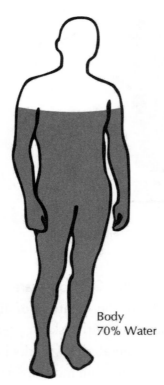

Body
70% Water

YOU ARE A BAG OF WATER

Our human bodies are **70 percent water.**[39] Some parts of our bodies contain more water than others. For example, your brain is 85 percent water, your blood stream is 83 percent, your muscles are 75 percent, and your joint cartilage is 82

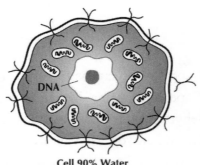

DNA

Cell 90% Water

percent.[4041] Your stomach lining contains the most water of any organ in your body; it's an amazing 98 percent H_2O![42] Most of your cells are about 90 percent water.[43] That's a lot of water! Look at the pictures to get an idea of how much water is inside of us. If you don't give your cells enough water, they shrivel up. They can't function correctly because water carries out many critical roles in your cells' day-to-day processes.[44] And when your cells don't function well, you don't function well.

If the water in your cells is contaminated, your whole body is contaminated. But don't worry: you have the opportunity to change things. Your cells are reborn every minute.[45] In fact, you won't have a single one of your current red blood cells in four months; they'll all be new.[46] Almost all of your cells live and die in a short period of time. Because your body is always changing, there's ample opportunity for you to improve it. Start drinking more water today and you'll feel the effects very quickly. Don't let another day go by living with shriveled cells. Drink plenty of good water everyday and you'll help prevent most sicknesses. Proper hydration can help alleviate the

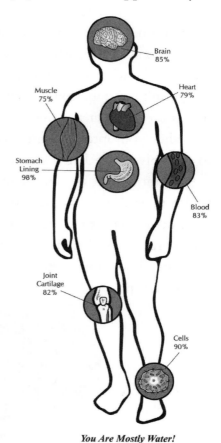

Brain 85%
Heart 79%
Muscle 75%
Stomach Lining 98%
Blood 83%
Joint Cartilage 82%
Cells 90%

You Are Mostly Water!

symptoms of asthma, ulcers, arthritis, herniated discs and wrinkles.[47]

YOUR STAGNANT WATER WILL DECAY

Drinking isn't something that will only help you in the abstract. On the contrary, drinking enough water will make a very tangible difference in your life. You've got to drink water all of the time so your body doesn't become a place where disease festers.[48] If you don't flush out your system with new water constantly, your insides become like a **pool of standing water, unclean and a perfect environment for toxins.** You don't want your internal water to be like this.

For good health, it's important to keep your body's water moving. As with a fast-running stream, moving water in your body can't build up toxins. Bugs like bacteria and viruses thrive in toxic environments that occur when water isn't flowing.[49] But when your internal water gets moving, they have no chance to multiply before being swept away.

And movement does more than just clean out our systems— it also nourishes us. Because of moving water, the cells in your body do not have to move to find food, as is the case with single-celled organisms. With us, food is brought to each cell by traveling water.[50] So, along with all the other benefits it gives, moving water feeds us!

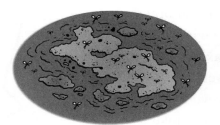

Stagnant Water Decays

It is estimated that we lose about 10 cups of water every day, even if we don't exercise.[51] Therefore, keeping our water flowing means drinking enough water to compensate for this daily loss. You've got to put in what will go out to stay healthy.

IF YOU DON'T DRINK . . .

If you don't drink enough water, not only will your body become toxic, but it will also suffer from dehydration. In fact, you'll enter what's known as the state of "**autointoxication**," an altered state brought on by too high a concentration of toxins in your body. In holistic medicine, autointoxication is considered the basis for all kinds of illnesses.[52] Just a few health problems that can be caused in part by insufficient water intake include asthma, high blood pressure, arthritis, ulcers, back pain, and wrinkles.

Sadly, **asthma** is one of the most common illnesses in North America, but a minor lifestyle change—drinking more water—can help prevent it. The culprit behind asthma is histamine, a neurotransmitter that regulates how water is distributed in your body.[53] When you're dehydrated, your body wants to restrict the water it gives to your lungs in favor of more vital organs like the heart and brain. This makes histamine production go up. And when blood that's concentrated with histamine reaches your lungs, it causes bronchial spasms, or asthmatic symptoms. These spasms are meant to preserve water in your body. So when you have an asthma attack, you're really experiencing an urgent need for water![54] If you drink the recommended amount of water—about eight to 10 cups each day for most people—many of your asthma symptoms will go away on their own.[55]

Another rampant illness is **hypertension**, or high blood pressure, which is also affected by dehydration. Every second of the day, your body takes water from your blood, filters it, and injects it into millions of cells all at one time. When there's not enough water available, this water exchange creates a rise in blood pressure. That's because your body, especially your heart, has to work harder to fill cells with water.[56]

Arthritis pain is yet another symptom of too little water consumption. Pain in your joints is an indication that there's not enough water in the cartilage of these areas.[57] The membranes on your joint surfaces keep the bones from rubbing together when you move. These membranes are 82 percent water. When you don't drink enough, your membranes shrivel.

Ulcers can almost always be linked to dehydration too. I've already mentioned that your stomach lining is 98 percent water. This mucous layer prevents acids associated with digestion from coming in contact with the walls of your stomach. But when you don't get enough water, your lining isn't as effective. It becomes thinner, allowing acids to get through and bring on stomach pain.[58] After a while, the acid will eat away at your stomach and begin to form ulcers.

Your **spinal joints** are made almost entirely of water as well, and a state of dehydration can affect them like it can most other parts of your body. In spinal joints, water lubricates contact spaces and fills the disc core. An amazing 75 percent of the weight of your upper body is supported by the water in your spinal discs![59] With so much pressure exerted on your discs, it is important that there is enough water present in your body to fill them. Otherwise, the hydraulic support system in your back will collapse, and pain will follow.

All the ladies reading this book will be interested in the next problem associated with too little water: **wrinkles**. Yes, dehydration can bring wrinkles too. When skin doesn't have enough water, it loses its color and elasticity.[60] As we age, we lose water content in our bodies. A young adult is made up of about 70 percent water, but by the time a person reaches old age, that percentage could be as low as 50.[61] The reduction in water is a big reason why the elderly have wrinkles. There's really no way to prevent wrinkles forever, but you'll do a good job delaying their onset with good hydration techniques.

DRINK BEFORE YOU GET THIRSTY

You have to be **proactive** when it comes to your health. You shouldn't wait until you feel thirsty to drink. Feeling thirsty means you're already dehydrated.[62] Drink before you get thirsty to prevent the effects of dehydration.

Water performs many key functions in your body; it plays a big role in energy production, activation and inhibition of reactions in the body, elimination of toxins, regulation of body temperature, and circulation of fluids.[63] Obviously, you need water to perform to your highest potential, but you aren't able to rely on your body to let you know when to drink. In fact, by the time you feel thirsty, you've already lost 2 to 4 percent of your body's water content![64] You might not think that's a lot, but a 2 percent loss is actually critical, especially when you consider that a 20 percent loss in water is certain death for most people.[65] If you lose just 1 percent of your total body weight in water, you could face a 10 percent loss in performance. And when 2 percent of your water is gone, a whopping 20 percent of performance potential leaves too.[66]

Next to oxygen, which we get automatically from breathing, water is one of the most crucial necessities for life, perhaps rivaled only by **salt**. I just told you that losing 20 percent of your body's water can lead to death. But you can lose half of your body's protein, fat, or sugar and you'll survive just fine. That should show you how important your water really is—lose just a little and you're in big trouble. Drinking before you're thirsty will guarantee that you won't reach dangerous levels of dehydration.

WATER DIET

Do you want to know the best way to lose weight? Just drink more water.[67] And go on a long walk. That's all it takes. Water can help you lose weight through its help in the activation of **lipase**, a fat-burning enzyme. Lipase gets "turned on" when you're active, but it needs water to help it work.[68]

Keeping hydrated will help you lose pounds, but not drinking enough water will have the opposite effect—dehydration leads to weight gain. That's because when you don't drink water, you cannot adequately retain sodium in your cells. The hormone aldosterone is released from the kidneys to increase sodium and water retention.[69] When you get too much of it circulating through your bloodstream, you will gain weight and your blood will increase in volume, hence your blood pressure will increase.[70]

The amount of water isn't the only thing that matters when it comes to your impact on the scale. The way you drink water can affect your weight too. You can't eat hot food with cold drinks; it puts too much stress on your body, and stress, as you will learn in detail further on, will always make you fat.[71] **Cold liquids** can be fine if you're overheated and need to cool down, like when you're exercising. But cold liquids mixed with greasy, warm food makes the fat in the food coagulate, which causes it to be absorbed more easily into your system. If, on the other hand, you eat greasy foods with warm liquids, like tea, you won't feel the ill effects as much. The fat won't be shocked by a drink that's similar to it in temperature, so you won't have coagulated fat floating around your system.

The Chinese know not to drink cold things with greasy foods. Their foods are just as greasy as many American staples, but since they always drink hot tea with their meals, they don't get fat and suffer as many heart attacks. Americans wash down greasy cheeseburgers with toxic, cold sodas—that's why we are overweight.

WHAT KIND OF WATER SHOULD YOU DRINK?

Processing is always bad, but you might not think about it when it comes to water. However, many of the waters we drink have been severely altered through chemical processes. And the more water is processed by man, the worse it becomes. Water has tremendous healing power, but this power is disrupted when it is processed.

Tap water is the worst kind of water to drink. It is full of **chlorine** and **fluoride**. These toxic minerals are added to kill pathogens, but they can also kill your cells. Chlorine and fluoride have been linked to heart disease and atherosclerosis because they scar the arterial linings. And when you have scarred blood vessels, cholesterol can build up.

Purified water should also be avoided. There are three common ways to **purify water**: distillation, deionization, and reverse osmosis. **Distillation** is one of the most common methods. It involves boiling water and then condensing the steam into a clean container, leaving most of contaminants behind. Distilled water is not good for human consumption. It is devoid of vital minerals, and its life force has been destroyed by boiling. **Deionization** is another common way to purify water. Deionization is a physical process that uses specially manufactured ion-exchange resins, which bind to mineral salts and filter them out from water. This process is a quick and effective way to remove all the valuable minerals from water, and it destroys all life energy. Finally, **reverse osmosis** is a purification method that uses pressure to force water through a membrane, retaining the minerals and allowing the water to pass to the other side. All the healing minerals are taken from water when reverse osmosis is used. Also, since such high pressure is exerted on the liquid, all the natural life force of water is destroyed.

Ionized water is my choice of liquid when natural spring water from artisan wells is not available. **Ionized /alkalized water** has been around in Japan since the 1950s. I have read numerous books in Japanese and Korean about the enormous **health benefits** of drinking ionized water. In the ionization process, water is split into positively and negatively charged panels through electrolysis. There are two types of ionized water that result: alkalized and acidic. The **alkalized water** is for drinking, and the acidic water is used for sanitation purposes. I have read books and seen actual footage on a large hospital in Japan, which treated diabetic patients with these waters. The patients' decaying ulcers were completely healed when the acidic water was used to soak the devitalized feet and the alkalized water was used for drinking. I will discuss this further in my upcoming book *9 Secrets of Healthy Feet*. I myself have been using an ionized water machine for more than 10 years now.

Natural artesian spring water is absolutely the healthiest water available. It has plenty of natural life-healing energy inside. There are many different spring waters available, but some are better than others. The quality of water is better when it comes from a more remote source. Fiji® water from the Fiji islands is 1500 miles away from major civilization. It also is in an **alkalized state,** with a pH of 7.5. The source of the spring is higher than 10,000 feet. The higher the source of water, the more healing power it has due to the levitation force that it accumulates when flowing against gravity. Any natural water from a high altitude source, such as the French Alps, will be healthiest to drink. Evian® water and Hawaiian water are some of the best waters available. However, many so-called "spring" waters are bottled at local areas. You should be very careful of these types of water.

CAFFEINE ADDICTION

Caffeine is the most popular **drug** on earth. It's in coffee, tea, cocoa, chocolate, soft drinks, more than 2,000 non-prescription drugs, and more than 1,000 prescription drugs.[72] Believe it or not, some form of caffeine is consumed by nearly 200 million Americans every day.[73] Amazingly, 100 million American adults drink three or more cups of coffee each day.[74] Tea and coffee are the top two beverages consumed on earth after plain water.[75] With that much caffeine consumption, it's clear that people are addicted. And this caffeine addiction is a huge epidemic in this country and in the rest of the world.

There are **three myths** surrounding caffeine:[76]

1.) CAFFEINE GIVES YOU ENERGY. Caffeine gives you just chemical stimulation, which is not true energy. Drinking a caffeine-filled cup of coffee or tea gives you some initial stimulation, but then it causes you to crash, which leads to **fatigue** due to increased stress hormones.

2.) CAFFEINE GIVES YOU A MENTAL LIFT. Drinking coffee or caffeinated tea won't make you happier in the long run. Caffeine does give you an initial lift in your emotions, but it ends up letting you down with **depression** and **anxiety**.

3.) CAFFEINE SHARPENS YOUR MIND. Drinking coffee won't make you perform better at mental tasks. You will feel increased sensation and activity at first, but the **quality** of your **thoughts** and your **recall** power will be decreased.

How do you know if you're addicted to caffeine? If you can't function without your morning cup of coffee, you are probably addicted. Similarly, if you drink multiple cups of coffee or tea throughout the afternoon to stay awake and alert, you likely have a problem. The true definition of caffeine addiction is this: you are addicted to caffeine if you have a craving for caffeine everyday and are consuming more than **300 mg** of it per day.[77]

Here are the caffeine values in tea, coffee and soft drinks.[78]

CAFFEINE VALUES IN TEA, COFFEE AND SOFT DRINKS

BEVERAGE	CAFFEINE (mg)
6 oz. instant coffee	100
6 oz. filtered drip coffee	150
8 oz. filtered drip coffee	200
12 oz. soft drink	40-100
6 oz. green tea	15-25
6 oz. black tea	50

SIDE EFFECTS OF CAFFEINE

There are too many side effects to mention them all, but I will go over the main results of a caffeine addiction below.

1.) ADDICTION. Regular use of caffeine increases the dopamine levels in your brain. Dopamine is responsible for pleasure and elation and is highly addictive. Cocaine and other drugs raise dopamine levels in the same way.[79]

2.) MALNUTRITION. Caffeine interferes with the absorption of vital nutrients in your stomach, including vitamin B, calcium, potassium and iron.

3.) INSOMNIA. Contrary to common belief, caffeine remains in your system for three to 12 hours after consumption.[80] A cup of coffee in the morning can keep you up later that night. The cumulative effect of this insomnia is devastating for your health. Caffeine messes up your sleep cycle, no matter which time of the day you have it.[81]

4.) LEARNING AND BEHAVIOR DISORDERS. Hyperactivity brought on by caffeine causes mood swings and attention deficit disorders. After lots of caffeine, you will eventually crash and will have decreased alertness, a shorter attention span, lower reaction time, less mental clarity, and a decreased energy level.

In addition to the main side effects of caffeine listed above, this drug can also lead to **fatigue, cancer, heart disease, stomach ulcers, headaches, allergies, PMS, birth defects** and **elevated blood sugar** levels. And that's just the beginning of it. Several more side effects have been linked to caffeine too.

Now let's talk more specifically about coffee. Coffee is an acidic beverage, and it's also a diuretic, which means that it eliminates more water from your system than it adds. In other words, drinking coffee will dehydrate you. If you have to drink coffee here and there, then you need to be responsible for your health and drink more water. I recommend drinking double the amount of water to compensate for the diuretic effects of coffee.

So if you drink a cup of coffee, then also drink two bottles of water to offset the dehydrated and acidic state of your body.

USE CAFFEINE WISELY

I myself don't drink coffee regularly. However, I do use coffee to my advantage when I need it. For instance, when I want to work out but feel too tired to make the effort, I drink a little bit of coffee. It enhances my metabolism and makes me have a great workout. Some days, I am too tired to clean my backyard or perform other household chores, so I drink a little bit of coffee to get me going. You can also use coffee or caffeine to your advantage if you consume it wisely. Only drink it when you need it. Also, don't drink coffee or other forms of caffeine every morning, especially on an empty stomach. This makes you gain weight around your stomach, and nobody wants that.

What are good alternatives to coffee and other highly caffeinated drinks? Clearly, the best choice is to drink water and only water. However, if you want another option, I recommend switching from coffee to tea drinking. **Herbal and green teas** have **polyphenols** and **catechins**, powerful antioxidants. Herbal teas have no caffeine, and green tea only has a small amount compared to coffee. If you insist on continuing with coffee, I recommend you drink organic kinds. Organic coffees are more natural and better for you than conventional varieties. I advise you to cut out soda and energy drinks altogether; these are no good. I will talk more about them in later chapters.

HOW ABOUT DECAFFEINATED DRINKS?

You might think that decaf coffees and teas are good alternatives to regular. However, this is definitely not true. Avoid decaf at all costs! Decaffeinated coffee or tea is **chemically processed** and is not good for you.[82] In addition, decaffeinated coffee still has plenty of caffeine in it. In fact, a 12 oz cup has at least 10 mg of caffeine.[83] That means when you drink five to ten cups of decaffeinated coffee, it is equivalent to drinking one or two cups of regular coffee in terms of caffeine consumption.

There are many different procedures that are used to decaffeinate coffee. These procedures are mostly synthetic and chemical processes that are harmful to you. For instance, one of the more common ways to make coffee decaf is to rinse the beans with methylene chloride for 10 hours, and then steam them for an additional 10 hours. All this processing may cause most caffeine to be removed, but it's just not healthy for you. Therefore, I recommend that if you still want to drink coffee or tea, drink regular rather than decaffeinated. Regular coffee is definitely the lesser evil.

IS ALCOHOL GOOD FOR YOU?

According to the Department of Health and Human Services, 68 percent of American males and 47 percent of American females drink alcohol occasionally.[84] Alcohol is both a stimulant and a depressant. It stimulates your brain cells but depresses your central nervous system.[85] Moreover, alcohol is a psychoactive drug that reduces your attention and slows your reaction speed. Some of the negative effects of alcohol include **intoxication, dehydration, alcohol poisoning, liver damage, brain damage,** and possible **addiction,** called alcoholism. Also, alcohol disturbs the sleep cycle. Many people have a "night cap" thinking that a drink before bed will help them sleep, but the opposite is true.

Despite the negative aspects of alcohol, there are plenty of benefits associated with an occasional drink, especially with red wine. Wine has phenols such as quercetin and rutin, and it decreases the clotting of platelets.[86] Many studies show that a moderate amount of wine—one to two glasses with a meal—can decrease your risk of heart disease, lower bad cholesterol, and decrease the chance of atherosclerosis, stroke, and kidney stones. One of the hottest topics about wine is its high content of **resveratrol**, a polyphenol compound found in grapes. This phytonutrient may inhibit cancer growth in humans and allow the cells to live 80 percent longer.

I love red wine with my meals at times. There are many health benefits of wine and other alcoholic beverages, but only when you use them wisely. A moderate amount of drinking in cultural and social settings can boost your circulation and immune system for positive health benefits. Just refrain from abusing it.

WHEN TO DRINK, WHEN NOT TO DRINK

Ideally, you should drink water about 30 minutes before you eat and again about 30 minutes to an hour after. Try not to drink with your meals; this will make you fat. If you drink before you eat, on the other hand, your body will feel satisfied sooner and you'll be less likely to overeat. A lot of times, when you think you're hungry, you're actually thirsty. Hydrating before a meal will teach you to distinguish between hunger and thirst.

I can't underscore enough the importance of **avoiding beverages while eating.** In addition to making you gain weight, drinking and eating at the same time will impede your digestion and absorption of foods. When you have a beverage with food, your digestive enzymes are diluted. This is especially true when you drink cold fluids with food; cold drinks not only dilute your digestive enzymes, but they also denature them. As a result of this enzyme dilution, you can't break down food very well.[87] You end up storing the food as fat. Also, your body doesn't get all the nutrition it needs from your meal.

I recommend drinking water throughout the day at set times. This way, you get in the habit of drinking before you're thirsty. Another way to get enough water is to just carry a large jug filled with your recommended water intake around with you. Sip on it all day and you'll get hydrated. I will go into further detail about when to drink in Chapter 10.

HOW MUCH WATER SHOULD YOU DRINK TO BE HEALTHY?

With all this talk about water, you're probably wondering how much you really need. That's tricky because exact amounts are different for every person. I'm sure you've heard that we all need seven to eight glasses of water per day; this is a good average number, but it's not accurate for everyone. I like to recommend that you drink half of your body weight in fluid ounces per day. If you're diabetic, however, you'll need to drink at least 100 ounces each day regardless of your weight. Anyone who wants to lose weight should drink more water too. More water equals more detoxification.

I also recommend you drink four times each day—once in the morning, once between breakfast and lunch, once between lunch and dinner, and once after your final meal. That's why we divide by four at the end of the following exercise.

EXERCISE: HOW MUCH WATER SHOULD I DRINK?

Your weight in pounds _____ ÷ 2 = _____ fluid ounces.

Convert _____ fluid ounces ÷ 16.9 fluid ounces = _____ bottles .

_____ bottles ÷ 4 = _____ bottles every time you drink.

Example: 150 pounds ÷ 2 = 75 ounces ÷ 16.9 fluid ounces = 4.4 bottles

4.4 bottles ÷ 4 = 1.1 bottles every time you drink

SCHEDULE YOUR HEALTH

Look at the chart below. The illustration on the left gives you an idea of when you should be drinking water; in the morning, between meals, and one hour after dinner. Fill out the chart on the right with your own water-drinking habits by drawing bottles at the times when you normally drink. How do you measure up?

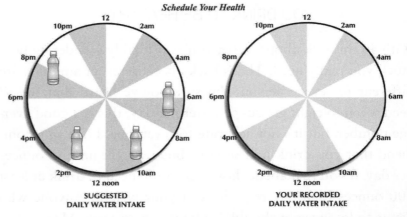

Schedule Your Health

SUGGESTED DAILY WATER INTAKE

YOUR RECORDED DAILY WATER INTAKE

WATER WELLNESS SCORING CHART

Use the following chart to determine how healthy your drinking habits are right now. Circle the kind of water you drink on the left side of the chart. On the right side, estimate how much you drink. If your answers fall above the line, give yourself one point. If they fall below the line, you're in trouble and get no points!

Water Wellness Scoring Chart
Circle what you drink and how much

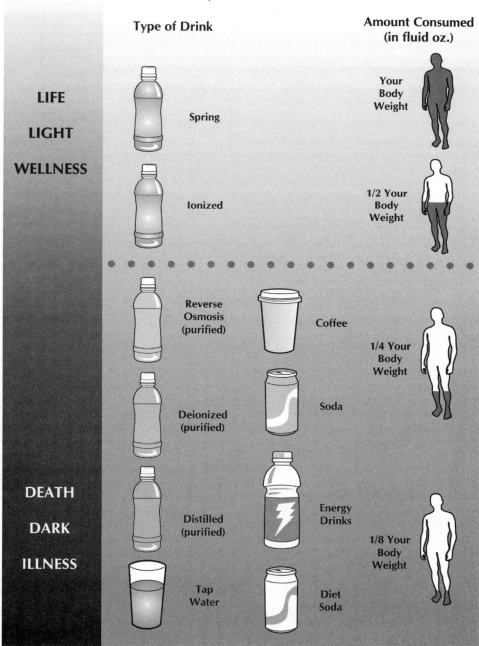

LIFE

LIGHT

WELLNESS

DEATH

DARK

ILLNESS

Type of Drink

Amount Consumed
(in fluid oz.)

Spring

Ionized

Reverse
Osmosis
(purified)

Coffee

Deionized
(purified)

Soda

Distilled
(purified)

Energy
Drinks

Tap
Water

Diet
Soda

Your
Body
Weight

1/2 Your
Body
Weight

1/4 Your
Body
Weight

1/8 Your
Body
Weight

Chapter 3

THE 2ND SECRET:
WOOD

"GREEN, GREEN, GREENS!"

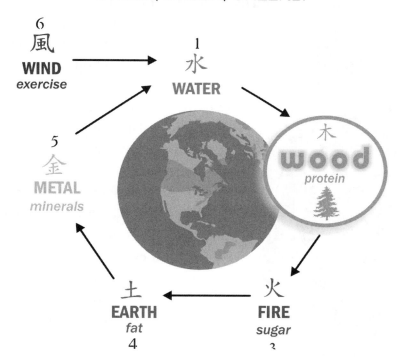

Our earth is covered with green trees that neutralize the toxic environment. Similarly, our bodies need green vegetables to neutralize toxins internally. Green vegetables provide us with all the necessary proteins that form the structure of our bodies. These greens provide enzymes that make our bodies work, balance our pH to heal all diseases, detoxify our organs, replenish our ever-needed blood, and allow us to lose weight healthfully by increasing our metabolism. By practicing "green, green, greens" daily, you will fuel your innate healing power to its full capacity.

YOU ARE MADE OF THIS STUFF

The term "protein" is derived from the Greek word "proteios," which means "of prime importance." And that's just what protein is—important. You owe a lot to protein. It's the **structure of your body**, upon which all other elements are built. Think of protein like the framework of a house: the frame is what supports all the other parts that will be added later. Look at the illustration of the human body. All of the parts shown in green are made of protein!

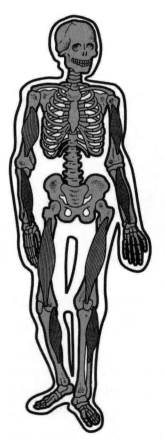

Structure of the Body

Protein makes up a big part of your **bones, teeth, muscles, enzymes, skin, and blood**. In fact, protein can be found in every cell of your body except in urine and bile.[88] The green parts in the picture of the cell shown on the next page represent protein. As you can see, your **DNA** itself is made of amino acids, which are the building blocks of protein. Proteins also can be found in your cell membranes, where they work as **receptors** and **effectors**. All cells of your body have **regulatory proteins** too.[89]

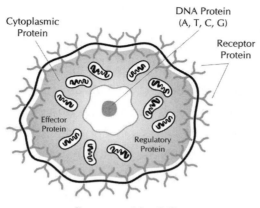

Structure of the Cell

Amazingly, there are more than 100,000 different kinds of protein in all of your cells![90]

What is protein anyway? That's a tricky question because there's no single "kind" of protein. In fact, your body makes countless proteins every day, and each one has a different function. Proteins are conglomerates of basic building blocks called amino acids. These amino acids can be put together to form different kinds of proteins. Your body needs 20 different kinds of amino acids, 11 of which can be made in your cells. But the remaining nine amino acids must be supplied from the foods you eat. These are called **essential amino acids**. All of the nine essential amino acids can be found in greens.

GREENS ARE THE BEST PROTEIN

Despite what you might think, **vegetables** are actually the best sources of protein out there. You probably envision meat and dairy products when you imagine where protein comes from. But while these sources are high in protein, they're not the best for you. That's because animal protein is processed; animals use plant amino acids to make proteins, and when we eat animals, we're only getting the protein that has been made more complex through this system of processing.

Plant proteins are easier for your body to use. A variety of greens can supply all that we need to make every protein in our bodies.[91] Greens provide you with all 20 amino acids, including the essential nine that you can't create on your own.[92]

Do you think you won't get enough protein from plants? Think again. Picture all of the world's biggest animals—giraffes, elephants, hippos, rhinoceroses, and gorillas. All of these creatures are herbivores; they don't eat meat. But they've still managed to find the protein needed to build huge muscle systems.[93] If the huge leaf eaters of the world can be strong and powerful eating only greens, you can too.

Becoming a vegetarian or vegan is a healthy option for everyone. However, although plants are better for you than animals when it comes to getting protein, you don't have to cut all meat products out of your life. I eat meat myself. But depending soley on meat products puts a lot of extra stress on your body. If you can't commit to eating only vegetables, you should at least try to make your diet more filled with greens. Change your perception of meat. Recognize that you don't have to eat meat at every meal to stay healthy.

GREENS HAVE LIVE ENZYMES

Enzymes are extremely important in your body. They start or speed up almost all internal chemical reactions, acting as catalysts to get your body working properly. Enzymes are like the builders of your body; they put all the proteins, fats, and carbohydrates together to make all of you.[94] And guess what? The great majority of enzymes are proteins.

Keeping a solid store of enzymes is critical for good health.

With the right enzymes, you're able to repair and recreate the parts of your body that need work. You can make many enzymes in your own cells, but you can also get them through the food you eat. Greens in particular are an excellent source of **live enzymes**. So when you eat plenty of fresh vegetables, you are helping your body fire up the chemical reactions that keep you going. And enzymes can keep you young too. Eating greens and the enzymes that come along with them can stimulate the production of **growth hormones** in your body. These hormones are necessary for vitality.[95]

The thing about enzymes, however, is they can be easily denatured, which means they will no longer work. Over processing greens through cooking can negate all the benefits of enzymes in these foods. Therefore, to get the most out of greens, you should eat them raw. Some cooking methods, like steaming, are okay too. Frying and microwaving should be avoided at all costs because these methods denature food. I'll talk more about how to cook foods the healthy way in Chapter Five.

GREENS AND PH

Liquids can be divided into two basic groups: those that are acidic and those that are alkaline. The graph that measures acidity is called the pH scale. It is a graph from 0 to 14, with seven being neutral. Just glancing at the pH of a liquid can show you whether it is an acid or a base. Any substance with a **pH of less than 7** is considered **acidic**. Anything with a **pH of more than 7** is considered a base, or **alkaline**.

It turns out that the most important measure of your health is the pH of your blood and tissues.[96] The **ideal pH for your bloodstream is 7.365**, which is slightly alkaline. But everyday, we add a lot of acidic chemicals to our bodies, such as food,

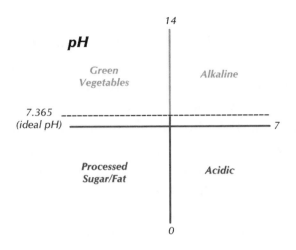

Balance Your PH

stress, and emotions, which lower our pH to unhealthy, acidic levels. And when your body gets too acidic, it gets sick. Acidity affects enzymes, which help carry out all the biochemical processes in your body. The toxins that swarm an overly acidic body weaken the ability to produce enzymes necessary for energy and organ activity.[97] Acid can also lead to a decreased absorption of protein, minerals, and other nutrients.[98] Too much acid makes you tired too, and it can make you more susceptible to allergies, colds, and headaches.[99] Eventually, cellular metabolism stops and your cells die. In chronic situations, you can die too.[100] [101]

Unfortunately, most people in industrialized nations suffer from overly acidic bodies. That's because most diets in these places are built around acidic foods, like sugars, carbohydrates, and animal proteins. In order to get our bodies' pH to its ideal level of 7.365, we need to balance out our toxic, acidic bodies with plenty of alkalizing green vegetables. We don't have to worry about getting too alkalized; with the amount of processed sugar and fat we eat, and the high levels of stress in our lives that won't happen. But by incorporating greens into every meal, we can raise our bodies' pH levels to the slightly alkaline 7.365. At this level, we function at our fullest potential. Diseases, which thrive in toxic environments, won't stand a chance. **Make your pH go up** with **green vegetables.** Don't let it drop too low with processed sugars and fats! I recommend testing your saliva or urine with a pH strip weekly.

GREENS BEFORE YOU GET SICK

A major point that I want you to remember is to be **proactive** about your health. I talked about this in the chapter on water, and I'm talking about it again now. You want to take a **proactive approach to disease,** warding anything off with healthy eating habits. Being proactive with greens means using them to create an alkalized environment in your body before you have problems with acidity. This will prevent health issues. If you keep a steady flow of alkalizing greens into your body, you'll balance out acidic foods and stress and maintain an ideal pH. And keeping your pH at its ideal level of 7.365 will proactively prevent sickness. So eat your greens regularly to stay well!

When should you eat greens? Get ready for it: you have to eat greens **at every meal.** This is why this chapter is called green, green, greens. And, yes, greens at every meal includes eating them for breakfast. In fact, breakfast is the most important time to eat greens because the morning is when your body is at its most acidic level. After a night of sleeping and detoxifying, you need two things: plenty of water and greens. This combination will neutralize the toxic acid in your body and will get you started on a productive day. Make sure you eat a breakfast that's high in protein and greens before you drink your morning coffee.

If you find it difficult to eat greens all the time, you could also purchase a mixture of greens to put in your water. I use an organic green powder called **"Green, Green Greens®"** in my water to make sure I get all the greens I need. I call the powder mixture my swamp water; it looks gross, but it's a great way to get all the greens you need and hydrate at the same time.

EXERCISE: PLAN YOUR GREEN-FILLED MEALS.

It's hard to know how to incorporate greens into every meal. Think about what greens you like to eat and write down different meal ideas. A few examples are given for you.

EXERCISE: PLAN YOUR GREEN-FILLED MEALS

It's hard to know how to incorporate greens into every meal. Think about which greens you like to eat and write down different meal ideas. A few examples are given for you.

Breakfast:
   Example: Omelet with fresh spinach, tomatoes, bell peppers and onions.

I would like to eat: _____

Lunch:
   Example: Mixed baby greens salad with tomatoes, cucumber, purple onions and carrots along with a healthy meat protein, like grilled chicken.

I would like to eat: _____

Dinner:
   Example: Steamed broccoli, cauliflower, carrots, pea pods and watercress with wilted mustard greens and fish.

I would like to eat: _____

GREENS KEEP YOU CLEAN

Greens pack fiber into every serving, and, as we all know, **fiber** helps with digestive health. They also help you detoxify, scrubbing away all the junk that's hanging around your veins and arteries and pushing it outside your body. I like to compare greens to a super scrubber for your bloodstream. They're a four-in-one cleaning tool for your insides, equivalent to a sponge, paper, soap, and WD-40®. Look at the illustration to see what I'm talking about.

Greens are like a **sponge** because they scrub away any buildup on the insides of your blood vessels with their high fiber content. If you eat enough greens—at every meal—you'll get all the fiber you need naturally. That means you'll have spick-and-span blood vessels. Greens are also like absorbent **paper**. They can wick away any bad fluids in your bloodstream. And they're like **soap** too. Soap cleans through alkalization. That's just what greens can do for your blood. Eating a diet filled with greens will cancel out the acidic effects of processed foods, cleansing your body of processed foods' acidic influence.

Finally, greens are like **WD-40®** because they are **natural antioxidants**. The amazing WD-40® prevents metal objects from rusting; similarly, greens keep your body from "rusting," or oxidizing, which is what happens when you age. In a way, greens reverse the aging process. **Oxidation** occurs when things get old. Atoms lose an electron to oxygen and are said to become oxidized. This is what happens when rust forms or fruit spoils; greedy oxygen takes an electron away from a substance and it ages. Think about a banana. It turns from green to yellow, and then from yellow to brown. Eventually, it shrivels up and turns black. Our own

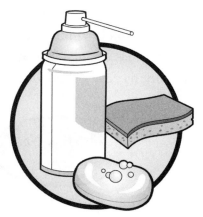

Greens Keep You Clean!

bodies undergo oxidation just like that banana, albeit at a much slower pace. Like the banana, oxidation in our bodies also leads to aging and other negative consequences. As antioxidants, greens can help reverse the oxidation process. The compounds in greens have an electron to spare, and they can loan this electron to your aging cells. So, in a way, greens can turn back time.

REPLENISH YOUR BLOOD WITH GREENS

As I mentioned in the introduction, you lose about 2.4 million (2,400,000) red blood cells each second. You make an amazing 25 trillion (25,000,000,000,000) red bloods cells every 120 days![102] Your body is replenishing blood cells constantly, and it's up to you to make sure it has the nutrients it needs to make strong ones. A large part of a red blood cell is **hemoglobin,** a substance that carries oxygen to all parts of your body. Did you know that **chlorophyll,** a pigment molecule found in plants, has almost an identical chemical structure as hemoglobin?[103] Like the picture shows, it's hard to tell them apart!

Eating greens provides your body with the building blocks it needs to make new red blood cells and replenish your blood stream. The exact relationship between chlorophyll and hemoglobin is unclear, but there is plenty of anecdotal evidence to suggest that eating chlorophyll-rich greens helps create healthy red blood cells.[104] And with all the blood cells that we lose every

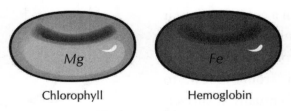

Chlorophyll   Hemoglobin

Plant Cell = Blood Cell

second, it's important that we do whatever it takes to replenish our supply—yet another reason for jumping on the "green, green greens!" bandwagon.

HOW MUCH PROTEIN DO YOU NEED?

You might be wondering just how much protein you need to stay healthy. According to the **World Health Organization**, men need at least **32 grams** of protein each day to stay healthy. Women need slightly less than this, except when they are pregnant or nursing.[105] Other sources recommend at least 50 grams of protein daily. Most people's palms are about 15 grams, so you need about three palm sizes. This will be discussed further in Chapter 10. Keep in mind that these are *minimum* values; you might need more protein to live optimally.

PROTEIN CONTENT IN FOODS

FOOD	PROTEIN (gms)	FOOD	PROTEIN (gms)
Peanuts (1 cup, dry roasted)	35	Potato (1 with skin)	5
Soybeans (1/2 dry roasted)	34	Mushrooms (chanterelle, 1 ounce)	5
Walnuts (1 cup)	30	Tomato paste (canned, ½ cup)	5
Pistachios (1 cup)	26	Artichoke (1 medium)	4
Quinoa (1 cup)	22	Avocado	4
Lentils (1 cup)	18	Dates (1 cup)	4
White beans (1 cup)	17	Hazelnuts (1 ounce)	4
Kidney beans (1 cup)	16	Prunes (1 cup)	4
Navy beans (1 cup)	16	Beets (2 raw)	3
Peas (split, 1 cup)	16	Corn (yellow, 1 ear)	3
Spirulina seaweed (1 ounce dried)	16	Fennel (1 bulb)	3
Yellow beans (1 cup)	16	Raspberries (1 pint)	3
Black beans (1 cup)	15	Spinach (1/2 cup)	3
Cauliflower (green raw, 1 head)	15	Beets (2 cooked)	2
Great northern beans (1 cup)	15	Asparagus (4 spears)	2
Lima beans (1 cup)	15	Beet greens (1/2 cup)	2
Pinto beans (1 cup)	14	Broccoli (1/2 cup cooked)	2
Sea cucumber (1 ounce dried)	14	Leeks (1)	2
Blakeye peas (1 cup)	13	Mustard greens (1/2 cup)	2
Cabbage (green raw, 1 head)	12	Papaya (1 fresh)	2
Chickpeas (1 cup canned)	12	Plantains (1)	2
Pecans (1 cup, halves)	8	Swiss chard (1/2 cup)	2
Pine nuts (1 ounce)	7	Tomato (1 cup fresh)	2
Squash seeds (1 ounce)	7	Truffles (1/2 ounce)	2
Fava beans (1/2 cup)	6	Brussels sprouts (1 sprout)	1
Figs (10 whole)	6	Carrots (1/2 cup raw)	1
Cashews (1 ounce)	5	Green beans (1/2 cup)	1
Eggplant (1 pound)	5	Mushrooms (Portobello, 2 ounces)	1
Lettuce (iceberg, 1 head)	5	Zucchini (1/2 cup raw)	1

You can read the labels of foods to find out exactly how much protein there is in each serving. If you look online, you can easily find the protein values for foods that are often sold without labels, like fresh vegetables.

Vegetables, nuts, and beans have plenty of protein. Look at the following examples to see just how much you could be getting from these foods.[106]

GREEN DIET

Did you know that eating greens can help you **lose weight** too? Proteins fire up your metabolism, getting your body to burn more calories. And burning calories is the way to lose weight. So eating greens can help you achieve a more slender figure.

Just from your own personal experience, you probably know that protein sticks with you for a long time. If you eat a protein-rich meal, your hunger will be satisfied for much longer than with a carbohydrate-filled one. With protein, you don't have to eat as often, which translates to fewer calories consumed. But protein does more than just satisfy your hunger. It also plays a big role in the hormones produced in your **thyroid gland**, which is the most important part of your metabolism. Your thyroid gland produces two nearly identical hormones that help regulate your metabolism: T3 and T4. T4 tells your body to reserve energy, thus creating fat. But T3 is more metabolically active; it tells your body to burn energy. Eating protein can help your body convert T4 hormones to T3s, which means that less of the food you eat gets stored as fat.[107]

The rate at which you burn calories, called your basal **metabolism**, is highest when you eat proteins. In fact, protein stimulates the metabolism by 20 to 30 percent![108] This is much more than carbohydrates, which stimulate basal metabolism by 5 to

8 percent, or fats, which only affect it by 2 to 4 percent. There's no doubt about it: protein is a weight-reduction food. When you eat protein, you burn more calories.[109]

Because of its significant effect on your metabolism, making proteins a bigger part of your diet is a good way to lose weight. And since greens are high in fiber, when you get your protein from plant products you'll have even more luck with weight loss. Fiber has been proven to promote weight loss and curb overeating.[110] Combine more greens with fewer carbohydrates and fats and you're well on your way to a thinner you. Green smoothies are excellent ways to get more greens in your diet. For smoothie recipes, I recommend reading *Green for Life* by Victoria Boutenko.

SCHEDULE YOUR HEALTH

Look at the chart below to see when you should be eating greens. As you can see, you need them when you first wake up, at lunch, and at dinner. A green snack, such as vegetables, fruits, nuts, and seeds, is good too. Now, draw in your green eating habits on the right side. How do you measure up?

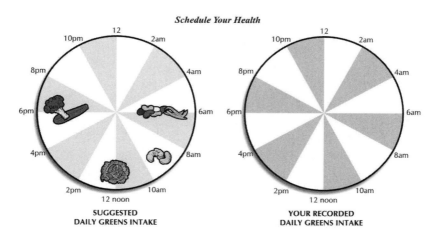

Schedule Your Health

SUGGESTED
DAILY GREENS INTAKE

YOUR RECORDED
DAILY GREENS INTAKE

GREEN WELLNESS SCORING CHART

The column on the left shows the greens that are good for you. As you can see, all fresh green vegetables and nuts are beneficial; the only bad greens are those that have been processed by canning, freezing, genetic modification and raised with pesticides and herbicides. Leafy green vegetables are at the top of the chart because they're best for you. Circle the greens you eat.

On the right side on the page, you'll see different cooking methods. Healthy preparations are on top and toxic ones are on the bottom. How do you prepare your food? Circle the methods that you use.

If more of your circles are above the line, give yourself one point. On the other hand, if you have several habits that fall below the wellness threshold, you don't get any credit. You should reevaluate your green eating habits.

Greens Wellness Scoring Chart
Circle what you eat and how you prepare it

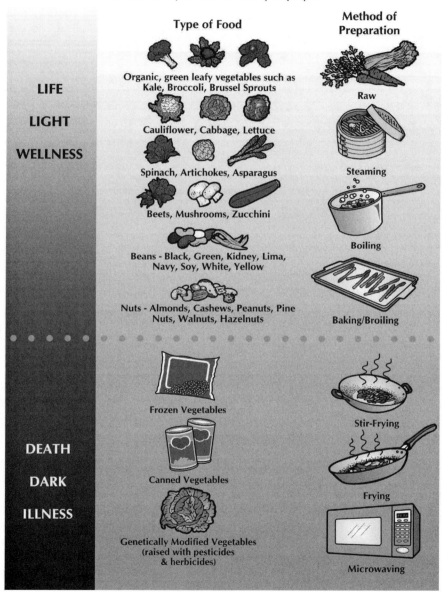

	Type of Food	Method of Preparation
LIFE	Organic, green leafy vegetables such as Kale, Broccoli, Brussel Sprouts	Raw
LIGHT	Cauliflower, Cabbage, Lettuce	Steaming
WELLNESS	Spinach, Artichokes, Asparagus	
	Beets, Mushrooms, Zucchini	Boiling
	Beans - Black, Green, Kidney, Lima, Navy, Soy, White, Yellow	
	Nuts - Almonds, Cashews, Peanuts, Pine Nuts, Walnuts, Hazelnuts	Baking/Broiling
	Frozen Vegetables	Stir-Frying
DEATH	Canned Vegetables	Frying
DARK		
ILLNESS	Genetically Modified Vegetables (raised with pesticides & herbicides)	Microwaving

Chapter 4
THE 3ʳᵈ SECRET:
FIRE

"REDUCE PROCESSED SUGAR"

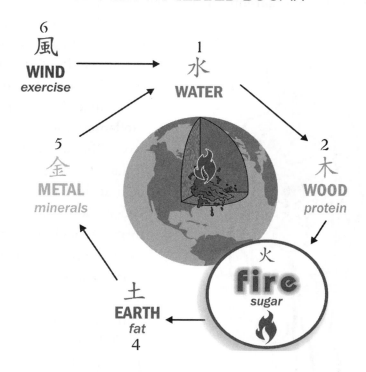

Our earth's core is made of fiery magma. Along the same lines, our bodies contain fiery sugar, which is the source of energy. However, when you ingest too much sugar, your body will be on fire with inflammatory diseases. Eating too much sugar will make you stiff, pollute your bloodstream, lead to addiction, make you fat, cause malnourishment, speed up the aging process, and reduce your healing power. By eliminating foods with refined sugar and increasing your intake of natural sugar, you will unleash the true power of sugar energy.

ARE YOU ON FIRE?

If you consume sugar products all day long, your body is on fire. You're not alone. Most Americans pack between 150 and 170 pounds of sugar into their bodies every year![111] That makes a lot of firepower. One of the ways this sugary fire manifests itself in your body is through chronic inflammation. After all, **"inflammation"** has the word "flame" as its root. In fact, sugar is the villain behind almost every "**-itis**" you could experience: arthritis, bronchitis, laryngitis, tendonitis, and many more. You can see this in the illustration. All of these "-itis" problems are based on inflammation, and all are caused by too much processed sugar.

Studies show that sugar could also contribute to more than 150 health problems, not limited to

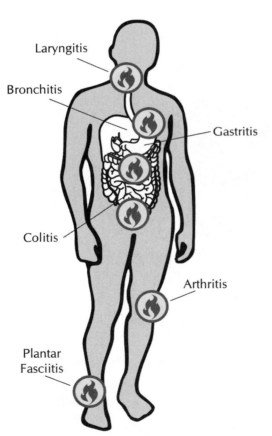

Laryngitis
Bronchitis
Gastritis
Colitis
Arthritis
Plantar Fasciitis

Your Body's Many Fires

obesity, diabetes, cancer, sexual dysfunction, and early aging. Sugar can also bring on emotional and cognitive problems like depression, irritability, forgetfulness, and suicidal thoughts.[112] It's terrible what sugar can do to you, and worst of all, it's scary to think that most Americans suffer from some sugar-related problems. We need to rethink our attitude about sugar to stop health problems from escalating.

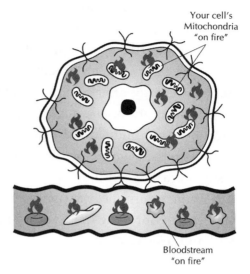

Your Cell's Many Fires

SUGAR IS THE GLUE THAT MAKES YOU STIFF!

If you've ever spilled a sugary drink on the floor, you know that sugar is sticky. Once the sweet liquid dries, it makes your feet stick as you walk over it. Even when you try to wipe up the sugary mess with a towel, you've still got a sticky floor to deal with. It's only when you scrub vigorously with water that the sticky sugar goes away. This sticky feeling isn't confined to the kitchen floor when sugar is spilled. Actually, sugar makes everything sticky, including your insides. Sugar becomes like glue in your body; everything sticks together and you get stiff.

You can think about sugar's effect on your body in terms of a hot volcano. The magma that spews from it is so hot that it destroys everything in its path. It produces a huge amount of energy through heat. But as soon as the lava cools down, it begins to harden. It forms a thick, gel-like substance that oozes over the land, finally solidifying into rock. Eventually, the lava forms new earth. This is just like what happens to our bodies when we eat too much processed sugar. We experience a huge burst of energy after eating something sweet. As you can see in the illustration, the sugar gets into your bloodstream and prompts your mitochondria to produce energy in overdrive. However, the sugar surge doesn't last for long. Soon, we have a sugar crash when the "heat"—or energy—of the sugar wears off. In the meantime, the sugar causes our blood to thicken and can lead to our own "new earth" in the form of fat. We end up stiff and overweight.

WHY DO YOU NEED SUGAR THEN?

With all the bad stuff that results from sugar, you might be tempted to avoid it altogether. But you can't do that. Not only would it be impossible to cut out all sugar from your life, but it also wouldn't be healthy to do so. After simple water, carbohydrates are the most widely consumed substance in the world. Glucose, the most basic carbohydrate, is the primary **source of energy** for most of your body. Your brain depends on glucose to function, as do your red blood cells.[113] In fact, blood sugar is the most important fuel burned in all your cells, including your muscle tissue.[114] Therefore, you can't eliminate glucose from your diet. You just have to learn to use it appropriately.

Our current levels of sugar consumption average out to about one cup of glucose per day for most people.[115] As I've already said, we need sugar to keep our bodies going, but one cup each day is way too much. Experts estimate that the equivalent of about **two tablespoons per day** is more in line with our needs. Anything extra contributes to the fire in our bodies, leading to inflammation, gelatinous arteries and veins, and an increased risk for disease.

NATURAL SUGAR, PROCESSED SUGAR

Natural versus processed sugar is the most important concept to learn when it comes to getting healthy with glucose. Natural sugar is good for you, but processed sugar is only out to wreak havoc on your life. I like to think of processed sugar in terms of the movie *Terminator*. The cyborg in that movie has no feelings for the human race because he is artificially made. Just like cyborgs, artificial sugars are out to kill us and create an artificial unhealthy environment in the body.

For your health, you always want to choose **natural sugars** over artificial or processed ones. Natural sugars are more complex. They take longer to be broken down and absorbed into your bloodstream because they have **fiber** holding them together. Processed, artificial sugars, on the other hand, are made so they can be absorbed almost immediately. They don't have any fiber in them. These carbohydrates spike your blood-glucose levels, causing you to feel a quick sugar high followed by a crash. What's more, processed sugars make you want more sugar all day to get back to the high, leading to a cycle of blood sugar spikes that can bring about all the health problems accompanying too much sugar. Processed sugars do nothing but create a disaster in your body. Unfortunately, about **85 percent** of all grain and sugar products eaten in America are extremely processed![116]

ARTIFICIAL SWEETENERS

Many people have recognized the problems that refined sugar products can bring about. But sometimes, they fight the sugar problem with an even greater hazard—artificial sweeteners. I will tell you right now that there's nothing good about any artificial sweetener on the market today. Anything made from a chemical process is toxic to your health; artificial sugars are more toxic than white, refined sugar, and they need to be replaced.

There are three main types of artificial sweeteners: aspartame, saccharine, and sucralose. These sweeteners are sold under the brand names NutraSweet®, Equal®, Sweet 'N Low®, and Splenda®. I will go into more detail about the toxic effects of these products in Chapter 10. For now, just know that they are all extremely unhealthy!

Besides their health risks, all forms of artificial sweeteners have been shown to actually increase cravings for sweet foods. They defeat their own purpose. People who use sugar substitutes want sugar even more! All in all, you'd be much better off staying away from sugar substitutes. Use **natural, organic honey, stevia,** or **agave nectar,** to sweeten your foods. All of these products come from plant sources.

ARE YOU ADDICTED TO SUGAR?

If you're a sugar addict, you should know that your problem isn't entirely your fault. Environmental factors such as the unending supply of processed carbohydrates and advertising campaigns for sugar-filled foods play a big part in any addiction. But chemical conditions in your own body could promote sugar addiction as well.

Carbohydrate sensitivity, low serotonin levels, and low beta-endorphin quantities can make some people more likely to be addicted than others. **Carbohydrate sensitivity** forces some people to experience more severe spikes in blood sugar when they eat sweet foods. They feel bad when their blood sugar drops, so they eat lots of sugar to keep it high. **Low serotonin levels** make people unable to pass up sweets. When it's present in normal amounts, the neurotransmitter is what allows us to forgo tempting foods. [117] People with low serotonin give in to their sugar cravings more easily. **Beta-endorphin** causes a feeling of euphoria. It's released when we eat sugary foods. People with low beta-endorphin levels experience extremely blissful feelings when they eat sugar, so they always want more. [118] For these people, sugar produces a high, just like highly addictive drugs.

All three of these problems—carbohydrate sensitivity, low serotonin levels, and beta-endorphin deficiency—can combine to make sugar addiction a very real problem for some people. Victims of sugar addiction can't pass up sweets, and when they eat them, they get a rush of energy followed by a terrible, debilitating feeling of withdrawal. As a result, they are like animals, constantly on the prowl for their next source of sugar. It's a miserable way to live.

SUGAR MAKES YOU FAT

Yes, processed sugar does make you fat. Since it's digested and absorbed so quickly, it's easy for your body to convert what it doesn't need into fat. **Insulin** is the hormone largely responsible for fat storage. Its primary job is to make sure your blood sugar levels don't get too high, and it does this by transporting glucose into cells to be stored as fat. When your blood sugar spikes, your pancreas releases insulin, sending your body into fat-storage mode. More complex carbs take longer to break down, so there's no spike, no outflow of insulin, and no fat conversion. Obviously, avoiding processed sugar is a good way to avoid excess weight gain.

It's clear that insulin isn't good for dieters. But there is another hormone that can help with weight loss. **Glucagon** acts as the opposite of insulin, working to raise blood sugar. It's sometimes called the fat-burning hormone because it stimulates the use of fat for energy. If you want glucagon to work, you cannot eat processed sugars. The only way glucagon begins to convert fat into energy is when there is not enough glucose in the blood as an energy alternative. Avoiding processed sugars stimulates glucagon release, and exercising can help kick it into action more quickly.

EXCESS SUGAR IS KILLING YOU!

Too much refined sugar won't just make you fat. It will also jeopardize your health! In many respects, sugar is a drug. Like any drug, it gives you highs and lows. It also upsets your body chemistry through a devastating chain of events. To start, **minerals are depleted** when too much sugar enters the bloodstream. Research has shown that excess sugar leaches the body of calcium. When calcium levels are low, other minerals become unbalanced too. Mineral deficiency ultimately results, and since enzymes depend on minerals to work, enzymatic activity slows as well. When enzymes don't work well, food isn't fully digested. The undigested food enters the blood stream, which alerts the immune system of a foreign body. The immune system expends energy removing the food, leaving the body in a weakened state. In the end, sugar leaves the body more susceptible to disease.[119]

Sugar not only **inhibits our immune systems,** but it also makes us less able to repair ourselves. Studies show that high blood glucose levels **inhibit the release of growth hormone.** And growth hormone is responsible not only for the obvious—growth—but also for important things like tissue repair, usage of fat storage, and metabolism boosting. To put it simply, growth hormone can help slow down the affects of aging. But when you eat sugar, your body doesn't release this important hormone, and you suffer the effects of an aging body.[120]

SUGAR DISEASES

TYPE II DIABETES is well known to be the result of a high-sugar diet. Diabetes begins as insulin resistance. At first, a person requires more and more insulin to get blood sugar back to normal levels after a spike. But after a while, no amount of insulin will clear the blood of its excess sugar. Eventually, the pancreas gets exhausted and stops making insulin altogether, causing full-on diabetes. If left untreated, diabetes can cause a number of larger problems like acidosis, coma, hypertension, shock, and even death.

HEART DISEASE is the single biggest killer of Americans, and it's strongly linked to high blood sugar. Insulin not only converts sugar to fat, but it also prompts the creation of cholesterol. And a buildup of cholesterol increases your risk of a heart attack.

HYPOGLYCEMIA is a condition in which the blood glucose levels fall below normal, causing sweating, anxiety, weakness, irritability, and drowsiness. When a reactive hypoglycemic person eats a sugary meal, he or she experiences a sudden spike in blood sugar, just like anyone else would. But in a hypoglycemic individual, the spike releases too much insulin, which removes blood glucose too quickly. The result is lower-than-normal blood sugar levels and a slew of undesirable symptoms.

POLYCYSTIC OVARIAN SYNDROME, or PCOS, can also result from insulin resistance, which occurs after regularly eating sugary foods. In PCOS, women develop multiple cysts on their ovaries during ovulation, which causes infertility problems and hormonal imbalances.

JACOB'S TESTIMONY

When my wife rolled me into Dr. Kim's office in a wheel chair, I was a mess. I had been a severe asthmatic for over 30 years and a diabetic for 2 years. I was on 13 medications, and had been hospitalized over 40 times. My blood sugar had gone as high as 600, which could be fatal for most people. I was taking seven shots of insulin daily, and barely keeping my blood sugar under control.

I met Dr. Kim after seeing 4 other surgeons, due to an accident at work. I was told I would be in a world of pain with arthritis for the rest of my life. Dr. Kim told me I needed surgery on my foot and ankle, but he wouldn't perform the surgery until I got my blood sugar under control. Dr. Kim asked me one question that started me on the road to recovery. "How would you like to be off all your medications?" he said. I didn't really believe that it was possible, but I was willing to try anything at that point. Dr. Kim told us about his seminars, and we agreed to go. At the seminar, a light bulb went off in our heads when we heard Dr. Kim speak. We had heard most of this information before, but Dr. Kim has a way of presenting information about health so that you can clearly understand it. He makes you see why you need to make changes to your lifestyle. After the seminar, we decided to give his program a try. We cleaned out our refrigerator of all the toxic foods. We started drinking our quota of water. We stopped all dairy products, drinking sodas and anything with processed sugar.

It was hard to stick to the program at first, but I was extremely dedicated. I started seeing changes almost immediately. I have now been off all my medications for over 3 years. Dr. Kim's program is nothing short of a miracle and I am living proof of a Life Transformed.

P.S. Not only was my wife able to get off her medications for thyroid and depression, she has been able to maintain a weight loss of 30 pounds.

COW'S MILK IS FOR COWS!

Most of us wouldn't consider milk to be a source of sugar, but it is a huge contributor to the sugar problem in America. By the time they are one year old, most humans are weaned from their mother's milk. Calves stop drinking cow's milk at around five weeks of age, as soon as they can eat grass. So why do grown-up humans still drink cows' milk, especially considering that cows' milk is different in composition from humans'?[121] Cows' milk is for cows only, and only very young cows at that!

When humans drink cows' milk, they get sick. It leads to terrible side effects, such as **iron-deficiency anemia, gastro-intestinal bleeding, bloating, eczema, cramps, diarrhea, allergies, asthma, atherosclerosis, heart attacks, kidney diseases, skin rashes, acne, leukemia, multiple sclerosis,** and **rheumatoid arthritis,** just to name a few. You might not want to hear it, but one of the best things you can do for your health is cut your milk habit! This includes other dairy products like cheese, ice cream, and butter.

Lactose is the sugar in milk. This sugar needs to be broken down into glucose and galactose to be used by your body. Unfortunately, many people do not naturally make lactase, the enzyme that breaks down lactose. If you can't break down lactose, you're said to be lactose intolerant. Lactose intolerance is characterized by stomachaches, headaches, and poor digestion after consuming milk products. Many people have a mild form of lactose intolerance and don't even know it. The condition is found in an estimated 80 percent of people of Asian descent and 70 percent of people of African descent. About 10 percent of people of European descent are lactose intolerant as well.[122] If about two-thirds of the world's population is allergic to milk, then clearly, cow's milk is really not an ideal food for humans.

The protein in milk is called casein. Humans are also highly sensitive to this protein. In addition, milk contains some of the most saturated fats around. Obviously, non-fat milk is a better alternative to whole milk if you can't get away from dairy products. Drinking a quart of whole milk means consuming 35 grams of fat, which is about 50 percent of your allowed fat intake for a day![123]

People ask me all the time, "Where do we get all the calcium we need without milk?" That is a great question. It is true that milk has about 1200 mg of calcium per quart. However, calcium is also in all dark, green, leafy vegetables and in broccoli, kidney beans, soy beans, almonds, seeds, and fishes.[124] You can get all the calcium you need from other sources.

PROCESSED MILK

Milk is bad enough on its own, but it gets even worse when it's sold commercially. In order to keep milk on the shelf longer, it is pasteurized and homogenized. Look at the picture on the next page to get an idea of these processes. **Pasteurization** kills all the microorganisms in milk, but this heating up to 280 degrees

Fahrenheit also kills all the live enzymes. This makes milk dead! After milk is pasteurized, it is **homogenized** to mix the cream into the liquid evenly. This is done by spinning at such a high speed that the cream is broken into small particles. These small particles are known to scar the lining of arteries, causing athero-sclerosis and, eventually, heart attacks. The processing of milk is absolutely devastating for your health.

As you can see in the next illustration, toxic, processed milk is then used to make yogurt, ice cream, and cheese. Therefore, all dairy products are bad for you. If you feel that you really don't want to quit milk, do yourself a favor and drink organic. I also recommend that you eat organic yogurt and cheese. If, how-ever, you have any symptoms that I described in the beginning of the milk section, please quit milk immediately. Oftentimes, quitting milk will completely cure people of chronic medical conditions, including asthma, allergies, and arthritis pain. A good alternative to cows' milk is **soy milk** or **almond milk**. I have been drinking almond milk for the last seven years, and it is nutritious and tastes great!

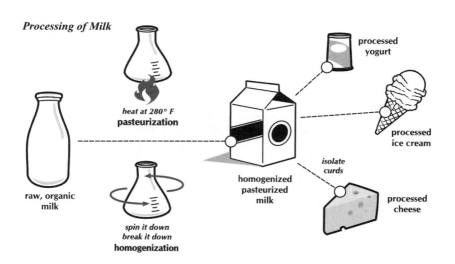

Processing of Milk

heat at 280° F
pasteurization

raw, organic
milk

spin it down
break it down
homogenization

processed
yogurt

processed
ice cream

isolate
curds

homogenized
pasteurized
milk

processed
cheese

Chocolate is another story. Many Americans can't imagine a world without chocolate, but it's actually incredibly harmful and addictive. Milk chocolate is not only heavy on the refined sugar, but it also contains drugs like caffeine, the stimulant theobromine, phenylethylamide, which is similar to the street drug ecstasy, and anandamide, a chemical related to the active ingredient in marijuana.[125] And of course, milk chocolate is made from milk, so you get all the bad things associated with the liquid when you eat it. Because of milk chocolate's high level of sugar and inclusion of so many harmful substances, it's best to stay away from it. If you are a certified chocoholic, try eating **dark chocolate** as a healthy alternative. Dark chocolate contains no milk, less sugar, is a powerful antioxidant, and has been shown to produce endorphins.

WHAT IS THE SOLUTION?

I've been talking all about how sugar can destroy your health. But what are you supposed to do about it? The solution lies in the **glycemic index**. The glycemic index (GI) measures how quickly carbohydrates are broken down and absorbed during digestion. The index is measured on a scale of 0 to 100 according to how quickly glucose from foods is absorbed into the blood[126]. Pure glucose is given an index of 100; it is the standard by which other foods are measured. Other foods are categorized as having

GLYCEMIC INDEX (GI) VALUES	
GI VALUE	**SCORE**
70 or Higher	High
56 to 69	Intermediate
0 to 55	Low

high, medium, or low GI values. You should try to stick to low GI foods for the best health.[127]

The following chart lists the GI values of some common carbohydrates.[128]

GLYCEMIC INDEX

CARBOHYDRATE	GI VALUE
Baguette	95
Cornflakes	84
Potato (baked)	84
Donut	76
Cheerios	75
Rice (basmati)	58
Muffin (bran)	56
Orange	44
Oatmeal	42
Spaghetti	41
Tomato	38
Apple	38
Beans	31
Yogurt (nonfat)	14

AVOID REFINED SUGAR FOODS

Refined sugar and foods that contain it have some of the highest glycemic indexes out there. Foods with high glycemic indexes can produce huge fluctuations in blood glucose levels, which gives you a burst of energy followed by a feeling of fatigue. You should cut the foods with the highest glycemic indexes out of your life altogether; they'll cause all the problems we've been talking about. Anything with processed, white sugar has to go. Foods with sky-high glycemic indexes include desserts like **ice cream, cookies** and **chocolate**. All of these sweet treats will send your blood sugar on a roller coaster ride and leave you burned out.

Bread products are better than sweet foods, but they're still full of processed carbohydrates. If you must eat them, limit how much you have and work out a bit more the next day. **Potatoes** and **rice** are filled with simple sugars too. Don't eat too many of these foods if you can help it. White rice and peeled potatoes are pretty much pure sugar; all the nutrition is in the skins or husks. So if you like potatoes, eat the skins too. If you like rice, try brown rice, which has the shells still attached. Eating these foods in their natural state will give them more of a nutritional value, although you should still avoid having them too often.

Pasta is surprisingly low on the GI scale. This may be because pasta is made of semolina, which is cracked wheat instead of finely ground wheat flour. But more likely, it's because of the network of gluten in the pasta, which has been shown to slow digestion.[129] Supplementing your diet with more pasta and fewer potato and flour starches can be a good way to fight excess sugar.

Although they can taste sweet, **unprocessed grains, fruits** and **vegetables** have lower glycemic indexes and are some of the best foods to eat. These foods are all complex carbohydrates, which means it takes your body a long time to break them down in digestion. They're also high in fiber, so they'll help clean out the bad stuff brought in with sugary foods. See the previous chapter on greens for more about fruits and vegetables.

GLYCEMIC LOAD

Clearly, the amount of the carbohydrates you eat will also have an effect on your sugar intake. That's where the glycemic load comes in handy. The glycemic load is a measurement that helps predict blood sugar response to a meal based on the type and amount of carbohydrates being eaten.[130] To calculate glycemic load, just follow this formula:

$$\text{GLYCEMIC LOAD}^{131} = \frac{\text{(GI value x carbohydrate amount per serving)}}{100}$$

Comparing the glycemic load of different foods will allow you to see which of these foods will have the most affect on your blood sugar. It's just like the GI, except that quantity is taken into account.

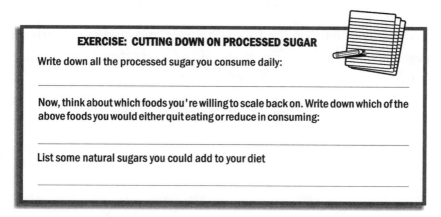

EXERCISE: CUTTING DOWN ON PROCESSED SUGAR

Write down all the processed sugar you consume daily:

_____

Now, think about which foods you're willing to scale back on. Write down which of the above foods you would either quit eating or reduce in consuming:

_____

List some natural sugars you could add to your diet

_____

SCHEDULE YOUR HEALTH

The chart on the next page shows the best times of day to eat carbohydrates. You need complex carbohydrates in the forms of fruits, vegetables, and unprocessed grains at every meal. You can also eat them for snacks. Draw in the carbs you eat and when you eat them on the empty chart.

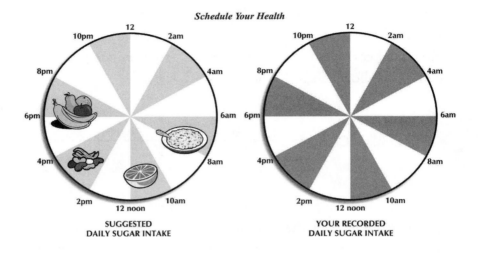

Schedule Your Health

SUGGESTED
DAILY SUGAR INTAKE

YOUR RECORDED
DAILY SUGAR INTAKE

SUGAR WELLNESS SCORING CHART

Look at the chart on the following page and circle the kinds of sugars you eat often. Give yourself one point if you circle more foods above the second dotted line.

Sugar Wellness Scoring Chart
Circle what you eat

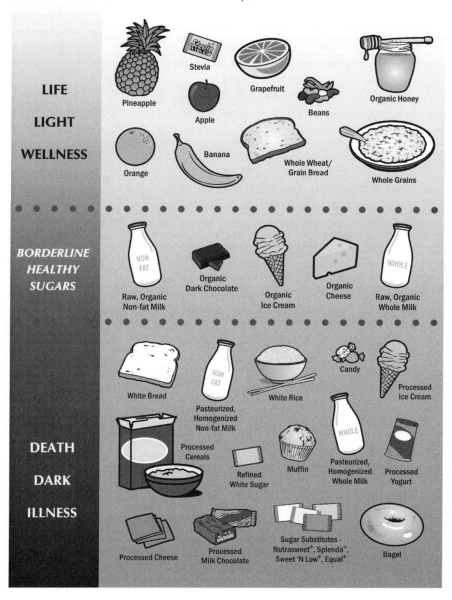

LIFE

LIGHT

WELLNESS

Pineapple
Stevia
Grapefruit
Apple
Beans
Organic Honey
Orange
Banana
Whole Wheat/ Grain Bread
Whole Grains

BORDERLINE
HEALTHY
SUGARS

Raw, Organic Non-fat Milk
Organic Dark Chocolate
Organic Ice Cream
Organic Cheese
Raw, Organic Whole Milk

DEATH

DARK

ILLNESS

White Bread
Pasteurized, Homogenized Non-fat Milk
White Rice
Candy
Processed Ice Cream
Processed Cereals
Refined White Sugar
Muffin
Pasteurized, Homogenized Whole Milk
Processed Yogurt
Processed Cheese
Processed Milk Chocolate
Sugar Substitutes - Nutrasweet®, Splenda®, Sweet 'N Low®, Equal®
Bagel

Chapter 5
THE 4ᵀᴴ SECRET:
EARTH

"INCREASE NATURAL FAT"

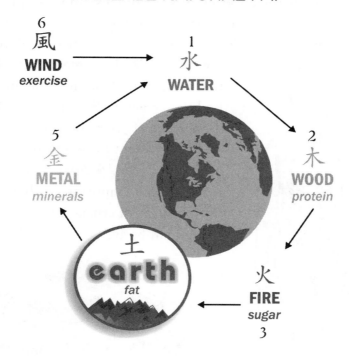

20 percent of our earth is covered with land. Likewise, 20 percent of our body is covered with fat, which is the bag that holds us together. Besides water, fat is the most abundant substance in our bodies. This is why low-fat diets are dangerous to our health; instead, we need to embark on the right fat diet. You need to eliminate

highly processed transfats and dramatically reduce your intake of saturated animal fats. You need to increase your consumption of natural plant fats to achieve true health. Now is the time for an oil change!

THIS IS WHAT IS HOLDING YOU TOGETHER

As you can see in the illustration below, fat is the substance that keeps your body's water intact. It holds the water within your cells, serves as the covering of your organs, and also provides outside support by strengthening your hair and fingernails. In fact, membranes made of fat cover every organ and cell in

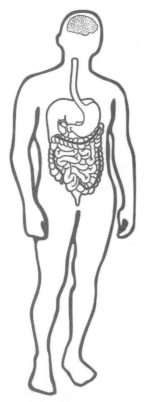

your body. With so many uses, fat is the most abundant material in your body after water. Fat makes up **15 to 22 percent** of your body composition, and it is present in two-thirds of your body's material.[132] Anyone who says that fat isn't important is lying—it's one of the most crucial components of the human body!

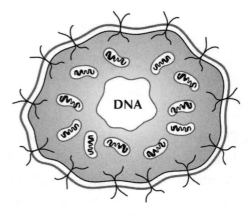

Your Body's Bag

The Cell's Bag

LOW FAT LIES

Did you think that fat was bad for you before picking up this book? If so, you're not the only person to have that misconception. However, research has shown that following a low-fat diet actually makes people fatter in the long run.[133] The low-fat diet doesn't work because it deprives our bodies of the most **vital material**—fat—that we need to rebuild ourselves.

When your body doesn't get enough fat from food, it begins making its own fat to compensate. What your body is doing is preparing for the worst-case scenario, a famine, but what you see is added pounds in the form of fat. And worst of all, the fat that your body produces while on a low-fat diet is one of the worst kinds out there—saturated fat.[134]

Despite what low-fat diet books may say, your diet should be at least 30 percent fat for the best balance. We will discuss exactly what kinds of fat and the correct combinations of these types at the end of this chapter. For now, just know that you need fat to stay healthy.

IS CHOLESTEROL THE WORST ENEMY?

No section on fat would be complete without a discussion of cholesterol, which is itself a kind of fat found in animal products. What do you know about cholesterol? You probably have been taught that cholesterol is bad, and that too much of it can lead to heart problems. This is partially true in that excess cholesterol can play a role in clogged arteries. But it's incorrect to think of cholesterol as a bad substance that you need to eliminate from your body. Cholesterol isn't the main culprit behind heart disease, although many people accuse it of being so. Actually, cholesterol plays a vital role in all animals, including humans, and you couldn't live without it. Cholesterol helps your body make **digestive enzymes,** plays a role in manufacturing **sex hormones,** and provides part of the protective outer layer on **nerve cells.**[135] It also helps make **vitamin D** and regulates all the **cell membranes** in your body.[136]

Although many people think that cholesterol comes from what they consume, this isn't true. In fact, your body produces most of its own cholesterol in your liver. For most people, only about 20 percent of cholesterol comes from outside foods; the remaining 80 percent is produced "in house," so to speak. [137] Another thing to know about cholesterol is that it can be affected by **stress.** Studies show that there's a correlation between repressed anxiety and high cholesterol.[138]

We are taught to think of cholesterol as a bad word, but really, it's a life saver. You need to have moderate levels of cholesterol in your body to function. But like anything, too much of it can have a harmful effect on your health. Over time, excess cholesterol can create plaque, which can narrow blood vessels and increase the risk of heart attack if left unchecked. But low cholesterol is just as bad. Too little cholesterol prevents your body from creating the hormones it needs to function and can prevent proper cell-to-cell interaction. Seniors especially need to watch out for low cholesterol because it can be very dangerous to their health.

INFLAMMATION IS THE CAUSE

In reality, **inflammation** is the cause of every chronic disease that's attributed to cholesterol. When your arteries become scratched and damaged on the inside, they become inflamed. Many substances, including cholesterol, come to the rescue to try to repair the hurt areas. Eventually, the cure becomes bigger than the original problem—cholesterol and the other substances build up in the arteries. Plaque grows and blocks blood flow, and, in time, can lead to a heart attack.

Many times, inflammation is aided with a buildup of **homocysteine,** an amino acid that is metabolized with the help of B vitamins. When your body doesn't have enough B vitamins to break down homocysteine, it accumulates in the blood. The lining of your arteries can become damaged and inflamed due to daily activities, and when homocysteine is present in high levels, this problem can worsen. The amino acid has also been linked to blood clot formation and the rupturing of plaque.[139] People who don't get enough B vitamins to metabolize homocysteine have a remarkable three times the risk of a heart attack compared to those who do consume these vitamins.[140]

As of now, there's no way for doctors to prevent damage and inflammation inside our arteries. But luckily, there is a way to find out if the inflammation is there or not. Measuring levels of a substance called **C-reactive protein,** or CRP, can show if arteries are inflamed, which helps establish if a patient is at risk for heart disease.[141] CRP testing is available in most cardiologists' offices.

HOW TO MAKE SENSE OF ALL THE NUMBERS

You've probably found yourself in the following scenario: you've just gotten your cholesterol test results back from blood that was drawn a few weeks ago. You flip through the pages of analyses, which are filled with numbers and acronyms like "LDL," "VLDL," and "TG." You think to yourself, "Great, I have my results, but what does all this mean?" I'm here to tell you.

Let's start with the basics—**LDL** and **HDL** cholesterol. LDL cholesterol, which stands for low-density lipoprotein, is bad for you. I call it the **"Lousy" cholesterol.** LDL cholesterol is produced in your liver and always makes up the majority of your total cholesterol reading.[142] LDL cholesterol is "bad" because too much of it can injure the insides of your blood vessels, leading to inflammation and buildup of plaque. For most people, a good LDL score is 100 mg/dL or lower.[143] **HDL** stands for high-density lipoprotein, and it's often known as "good" cholesterol. I call it **"Happy" cholesterol**. Like LDL, HDL is manufactured in the liver, but it's also made in the intestines and other parts of your body.[144] HDL seeks out damaged cholesterol—usually of the LDL variety—and brings it back to the liver for reuse, excretion, or processing.[145] For most people, a good HDL score is above 40 mg/dL, and any score above 60 mg/dL is excellent. A diet with plenty of good fat, like olive oil, is the best way to up your HDL.[146]

A good way to determine if you have enough HDL cholesterol in your body is to figure out your **total cholesterol to HDL ratio**. Just use the following equation to figure out your personal ratio:

$$\frac{\text{Total Cholesterol}}{\text{HDL Cholesterol}} = \text{Ratio}$$

A ratio of more than four is dangerous. It usually means that you don't have enough HDL to clear out your arteries of clogging agents, like LDL. Any number lower than four is good, but a score of three or lower is even better.[147] If you have a high ratio, you are at a higher risk of heart disease.

Another lipoprotein reading that shows up on blood test results is **VLDL**, which stands for very low-density lipoprotein. VLDL transports triglycerides, or fats, from the liver to other organs in the body. After VLDL drops its fat, it breaks down to become LDL. Usually, VLDL is incorporated into your total triglyceride number, which should be less than 150 mg/dL for good health.[148] Those **triglycerides,** which are sometimes abbreviated TGs, are the main kind of fat found in your body. They are also present in most fats and oils that you eat. Like cholesterol, TGs perform many crucial functions in your body; they provide insulation, protect delicate muscles and nerves, store energy for future use, and fuel most of your body's organs. But excess triglycerides in your blood can damage arteries, leading to heart disease.[149]

THE GOOD, THE BAD, AND THE UGLY

Read over my list of good, bad, and ugly fats to learn what to include and avoid in your diet. The picture on the next page will show you how each fat looks in chemical form.

Good fats are those that are unsaturated, which are harder for your body to break down than saturated fats. There are two types of unsaturated fats: monounsaturated fats and polyunsaturated fats. Monounsaturated fats are almost always good for you; they are found in **olive oil, canola oil,** and **avocadoes,** and have been shown to reduce the risk of metabolic disorders and cancer. I've named these fats **Magnificent Monounsaturated Fats** because they are so good for you.

Polyunsaturated fats are more complicated as far as your health is concerned. These fats, known as omega fatty acids, come in two forms—omega-3 fatty acids and omega-6s.[150] Omega-3s are good fats because they can improve your heart's health and have been linked to a lower risk of cancer. I like to call these fats **Omnipotent Omega-3s** because they can help all aspects of your health. Omega-6s are important too, and they can help lower blood cholesterol levels. But omega-6s can cause harm if eaten in abundance; in fact, some researchers blame

TYPES of FAT

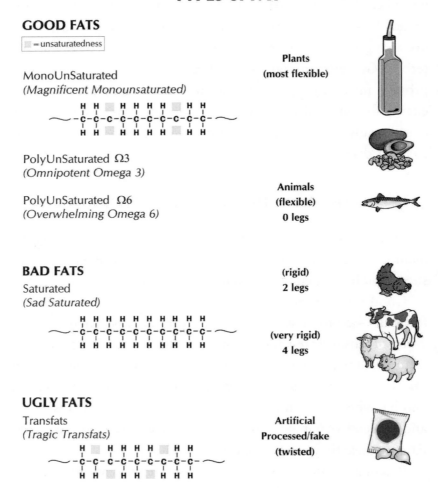

GOOD FATS

= unsaturatedness

Plants
(most flexible)

MonoUnSaturated
(Magnificent Monounsaturated)

PolyUnSaturated Ω3
(Omnipotent Omega 3)

Animals
(flexible)
0 legs

PolyUnSaturated Ω6
(Overwhelming Omega 6)

BAD FATS

Saturated
(Sad Saturated)

(rigid)
2 legs

(very rigid)
4 legs

UGLY FATS

Transfats
(Tragic Transfats)

Artificial
Processed/fake
(twisted)

problems such as cancer, allergies, heart disease, and asthma on too many omega-6s in diets.[151] For this reason, I call them **Overwhelming Omega-6s** because you can easily get too many of them.

Another bad fat is saturated fat, which is found in animal products like fatty meat, butter, eggs, and whole milk. Saturated fat can raise your LDL cholesterol levels, and it may increase your blood pressure and up your risk of blood clots.[152] For these reasons, I've named this group **Sad Saturated Fats**. Saturated fats are processed—they are created when animals use plant fats to create their own fat stores. It can be difficult to cut all saturated fat out of your diet, but scaling back on fatty animal products will decrease your consumption of them and improve your health.

TRANSFAT: THE ULTIMATE VILLAIN

Now onto the ugly: **transfats**. Nothing good comes of these fats, which can be found in most snack foods with a long shelf life. They are overly processed and are related to almost every health problem, including cancer. I call these fats **Tragic Transfats** because they can destroy your health. Tragic Transfats have been shown to lower HDL and raise LDL, which is the worst combination of effects possible. They can also interfere with cell chemistry. But despite all the bad things that come from trans-fats, people eat them every day. Unfortunately, most Americans eat five to 10 percent of their calories from trans-fatty acids, and many of these people have no idea how bad they are or where they can be found.[153]

Transfats became popular in the middle 20th century as a way to prolong the shelf life of foods. These kinds of fats are a result of **hydrogenation,** a chemical process which transforms vegetable oil into a solid substance. When hydrogenated oils are added to foods, they preserve them for months without refrigeration. Most foods with a long shelf life, including most snack foods, contain partially hydrogenated oils, the euphemism for transfats. These terrible fats can also be found in many fast food meals, store-bought bakery items, artificial cheeses, and margarine.[154]

Since 2006, producers have been required to list the amount of transfats in a product along with other nutritional facts. Usually, this number can be found underneath the heading for total fat grams. It's important to know, however, that manufacturers aren't required to list transfats if they amount to less than one gram per serving. Therefore, many products that contain transfats aren't clearly marked as having them. When in doubt, read the ingredients on a package; if the words "**partially hydrogenated**" appear, transfats are inside.

THE FEWER LEGS THE BETTER

A good rule of thumb when it comes to finding good fat is to look to the legs. Animals with multiple legs tend to provide the worst kinds of fats. Beef, lamb, pork, and other four-legged creatures offer meat that's high in saturated fat and bad to eat on a regular basis. Two-legged animals, like chicken and turkey, are much better to eat. The best fats of all, however, come from legless foods. Fish and other seafood products are excellent sources of omega-3 fatty acids. And, in general, plant fats are best for you too. The trick to plant fats is to avoid tropical plant oils, like those that come from coconut and palm, because they are high in saturated fats.

HOW ABOUT EGGS?

Many diet programs say that eggs are very bad for you because they are packed with cholesterol. However, eggs can be an excellent source of good fats, including omega -3 fatty acids. Look for **free-range eggs** for the best fat content; free-range eggs have an amazing 1:1 ratio of omega-3 to omega-6 fats! Store brand eggs, on the other hand, have a 1:20 ratio.[155]

If you don't want to down a full 212 mg of cholesterol when you eat an egg, leave out the yolk. Egg whites by themselves are an ideal food, with high amounts of protein, low cholesterol, and no saturated fat.[156] The yolks are where the bad stuff can be found. Yolks are high in cholesterol and should be avoided by people with heart problems or cholesterol issues. But if you don't have health problems, eat a few yolks now and then. They are an excellent source of lecithin, a substance that can aid digestion, enhance brain function, and can improve heart health. In fact, lecithin helps to regulate the transfer of cholesterol, so it almost cancels out any of the bad effects of egg yolks.[157]

HEALTHY AND UNHEALTHY COOKING

There are many options when it comes to cooking fats, and some are healthier than others. It's good to use the rule of processing when you decide how to prepare your foods. Based on this rule, **microwaving** is the worst. When the temperature rises very quickly as with microwaving, it denatures all the living things in foods. After much research, Russians banned the usage of microwave throughout the whole country due to its cancer causing abilities. It should never be used! **Frying** is another cooking choice that you should always avoid. When you fry a food, it completely denatures all the good stuff in it also. Even if healthy oils are used in frying, they are made toxic by the rapid oxidation that takes place when the fat is subjected to high heat, light, and oxygen. Most of the health benefits of foods are lost in frying.[158]

A healthy alternative to frying is **boiling** in water. When a food is boiled, its temperature cannot rise past the boiling point of water at 100 degrees Celsius, so most of the valuable nutrients and oils remain intact. Even sensitive oils like omega-3s can withstand boiling temperatures. **Baking** is another cooking option that can be acceptable for foods, although it's not as good as boiling. When foods are baked, they are exposed to higher temperatures on their outside, denaturing some of the valuable oils inside too.[159]

It's best if you avoid processing your foods altogether. Eat good fats in the form of nuts, oils, and avocados. Sushi can be an excellent, unprocessed way to eat fish too. It probably won't be feasible for you to eat all your good fats **raw**, but making an effort to incorporate less processing into your diet will make a big difference in the fats' nutritional values. **Steaming** is a good cooking method too.

EXCESS FAT IS A TOXIC WASTE DUMP

Belly fat isn't meant to hold up your pants. It's actually a toxic waste dump for your body, a place where all the unwanted waste accumulates. Many chemicals that have become a part of our lives over the last century are fat soluble, which means they can be stored in fat tissue. So your spare tire could be storing things like pesticides, flame retardants, dioxins, and plasticizers![160]

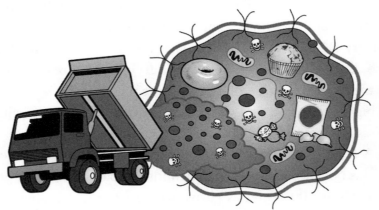

Fat Cell is a Toxic Waste Dump

Look at the illustration on the previous page to get an idea of what bad fat does to your cells.

If left unchecked, excess fat with **stores of toxins** can cause inflammation of the organs, which can lead to disease. The toxins get into your blood stream and cause all sorts of problems. When toxic fat interacts with organs via the blood long enough, it leads to a breakdown in the immune system. Allergies, asthma, cancer, inflammation, neurological disorders, diabetes, and autoimmune diseases can all result from accumulated toxins that migrate to the bloodstream from stored fat.[161]

IT'S TIME FOR AN OIL CHANGE

For the best health, you need to change the kinds of fats and oils you put into your body. **Omega-3 fatty acids** are what you need to keep moving. But unfortunately, omega-3s have fallen out of favor in most Western diets. Foods that are high in omega-3s, like fish and walnuts, tend to **spoil quickly** and cost more than their processed, trans-fat-laden counterparts. Most Americans only eat these good foods sparingly, and some avoid them altogether. In fact, nowadays, we eat an incredible amount of fat, but not the good fat that we need for health.

Omega-3s are super foods, and everyone would benefit from shaping their diet to mimic the ideal omega ratio. Omnipotent omega-3s provide multiple health benefits; in addition to their effects on cholesterol, which I've already mentioned, omega-3s can fight off cancer, improve metabolism, boost your immune system, and even ward off depression and other mental disorders.[162] Foods like fish, flax seeds, and walnuts are excellent sources of omega-3s, as are some dark, leafy greens. Incorporating oils with omega-3s into your diet can help improve your omega ratio too; flaxseed, walnut, canola, and soybean oils all provide significant amounts of omega-3 fatty acids. Meats and dairy products fall into the omega-6 category and should be eaten only sparingly.

The ideal **ratio of omega-3s and omega-6s is 1:4.** Unfortunately, most Americans have a ratio of 1:20. Some studies show up to 1:100. This is outrageous! This is why we are unhealthy and sick. I call a diet rich in omega-3 fats the **right fat** diet. It includes a balanced ratio of fats to help keep you healthy. On the **right fat** diet, you not only have to increase your consumption of omega-3 fatty acids, but you also have to cut down saturated fats and eliminate transfats from your life. With this combination, you'll experience the many benefits of omega-3s without getting bogged down in toxic fat.

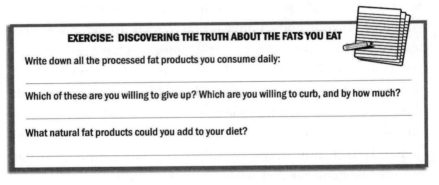

EXERCISE: DISCOVERING THE TRUTH ABOUT THE FATS YOU EAT

Write down all the processed fat products you consume daily:

_____

Which of these are you willing to give up? Which are you willing to curb, and by how much?

_____

What natural fat products could you add to your diet?

_____

SCHEDULE YOUR HEALTH

Look at the chart on the next page to see when you should be eating healthy fats. Then, pencil in the fats you eat during an average day. How do you compare to the ideal?

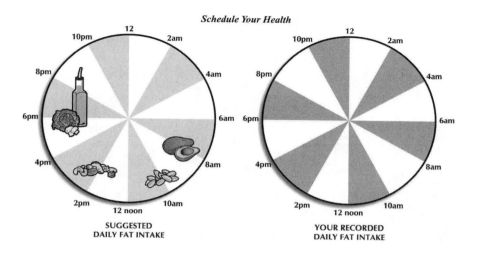

Schedule Your Health

SUGGESTED
DAILY FAT INTAKE

YOUR RECORDED
DAILY FAT INTAKE

FAT WELLNESS SCORING CHART

The illustration on the next page shows the good, the bad, and the ugly. Good fats are in the top third of the page. Okay fats are in the middle. The fats on the bottom are bad. Circle the fats and cooking methods you use most often. Give yourself one point if more of your circles fall in the top two-thirds of the chart.

Fat Wellness Scoring Chart
Circle what you eat

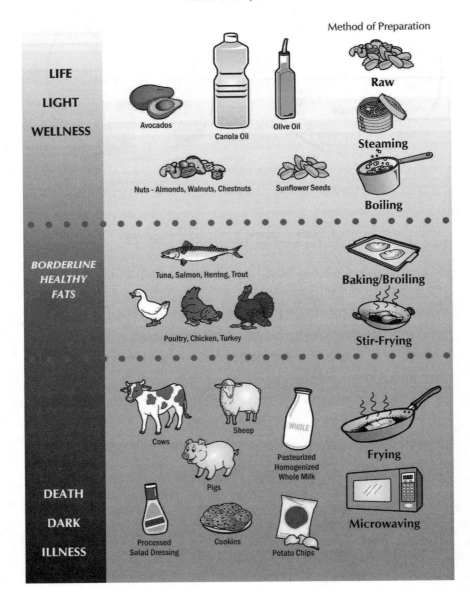

Method of Preparation

LIFE

LIGHT

WELLNESS

Avocados

Canola Oil

Olive Oil

Raw

Steaming

Nuts - Almonds, Walnuts, Chestnuts

Sunflower Seeds

Boiling

BORDERLINE HEALTHY FATS

Tuna, Salmon, Herring, Trout

Poultry, Chicken, Turkey

Baking/Broiling

Stir-Frying

Cows

Sheep

Pigs

Pasteurized Homogenized Whole Milk

Frying

DEATH

DARK

ILLNESS

Processed Salad Dressing

Cookies

Potato Chips

Microwaving

Chapter 6
THE 5ᵀᴴ SECRET:
METAL

"SUPPLEMENT VITAMINS & MINERALS DAILY"

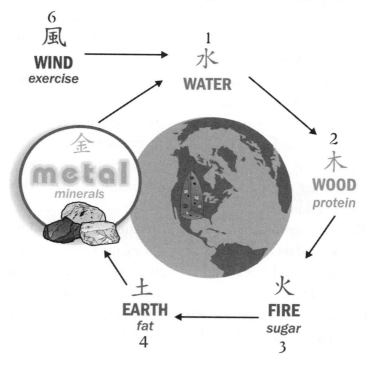

2 to 4 percent of our earth is embedded with metals. Metal is crucial for life on earth. Similarly, 2 to 4 percent of our bodies are minerals, and a proper balance of these minerals is essential for our health. With depleted soil and poor diets, we aren't getting enough of the essential nutrients we need to stay healthy. We need to supplement

vitamins, minerals, phytonutrients, antioxidants, probiotics, and digestive enzymes to make our bodies work optimally. The most important mineral of all is unrefined natural salt.

YOU ARE MALNOURISHED

It's not only happening in Africa and Asia. **Malnourishment** is a big problem close to home too. In fact, you are more than likely malnourished yourself. Even if you eat all the right foods everyday, you probably aren't getting all the vitamins and minerals you need. That's because most of our commercial food supplies in North America no longer contain the nutrients your body needs to work properly.

Unfortunately, the over farming of our land and the use of chemical pesticides has led to a depletion of most of the earth's natural minerals. The soil that was once fruitful is now dead because we used it too much. And the use of chemical pesticides has only made the situation worse; now, not only is the soil depleted of good minerals, but it's also filled with toxic chemical additives.

Farmers no longer use natural fertilizers that could replenish the soil of its minerals. Instead, they infuse it with nitrogen, phosphorus, and potassium, or NPK, the three minerals that plants need to grow.[163] All other nutrients are ignored. Now, the only way for us to get the variety of nutrients we need is with regular vitamin and mineral supplements.[164]

THE WORLD IS DEPLETED

All over the world, soils have been leached of their mineral content over the last 100 years. But North American soils are the worst of all. According to a 1992 Earth Summit Report, North

MINERAL DEPLETION OF CONTINENTS OVER THE LAST 100 YEARS	
CONTINENT	**PERCENTAGE**
North America	85
South America	76
Asia	76
Africa	74
Europe	72
Australia	55

America lost 85 percent of its soils' nutrients in the last century.[165] It's been almost 20 years since that research has been done, and the results don't appear to be getting better. Then and now, North America is far more affected by soil inadequacies than other continents. [166]

When there's nothing good in the ground where food is grown, there's nothing good in the plants either. And many of the vitamins and minerals that can be found in foods are denatured when these foods are processed, cooked, and stored.[167] That means the scant vitamins that we do get from foods very rarely make it into our bodies. To make matters worse, the toxic environment that surrounds us these days means that we need more nutrients to stay healthy.[168] In addition, if you maintain a stressful lifestyle or cope with chronic disease, you need even more vitamins and minerals than you would otherwise.[169]

OTHER REASONS FOR MALNOURISHMENT

Another devastating fact about nutrition is that more than 100 million Americans have problems with **digestion**. Even if they do get all the vitamins and minerals they need, their bodies can't absorb them. The main reason behind digestive issues is a lack of **hydrochloric acid** and scarcity of **digestive enzymes**, which work to break down food in the stomach, small intestines, and large intestines.[170] Certain allergies and digestive diseases can hinder the breakdown and absorption of foods as well. For example, celiac disease can change the lining of the small intestine, preventing proper digestion. This problem can be caused by mild allergies to milk, soy, wheat, and other grains.[171]

Medications can also sabotage the uptake of nutrients, and research shows that 19 of the 25 most commonly prescribed drugs could affect your body's ability to absorb vitamins and minerals.[172] For example, antacids may interfere with the absorption of calcium, copper, and folate; antibiotics could prevent magnesium, potassium, and calcium from being absorbed; high blood pressure medication may adversely affect levels of vitamin B_6; and common anti-inflammatory agents, like aspirin, could prevent proper uptake of vitamin C, iron, and folate.[173]

In general, Americans are deficient in the following vitamins and minerals. As you can see from the table below, some nutrient deficiencies are more of a problem than others. [174]

VITAMIN & MINERAL DEFICIENCY											
VITAMIN OR MINERAL	A	B	C	D	E	K	CALCIUM	MAGNESIUM	POTASSIUM	IRON	COPPER	ZINC
PERCENT OF AMERICANS DEFICIENT	44	28	31	20	93	73	75	56	95	20	25	30

YOU NEED TO SUPPLEMENT TO COMPLEMENT

The vitamins and minerals listed in the table above aren't the only nutrients you need to stay healthy. Actually, you need to give your body a total of 88 essential nutrients that you can't produce on your own. These essential nutrients include 60 minerals, 16 vitamins and phytonutrients, nine amino acids, and three fatty acids.[175] These vitamins and minerals make your body work.

You should do all that you can to get essential nutrients from foods by eating healthy, well-balanced meals. After all, no amount of supplementing can replace the way a great meal makes you feel. But since there's no way you'll get all the nutrients you need from food alone, you need to take supplements to complement food. In fact, the October 2002 edition of the *Journal of the American Medical Association* reported that every adult should supplement because it has become impossible to get essential nutrients through diet alone.[176]

If you don't get all of the essential nutrients your body needs, then you will be at a high risk of contracting the following diseases. Supplementing is a good way to ward off many of these problems. [177]

These diseases aren't the only problems you'll face if you aren't providing your body with the vitamins and minerals it needs. Calcium deficiency alone can cause 147 diseases, most of which aren't listed below![178]

THE NEED FOR MINERALS

ILLNESS	DEFICIENCY
Osteoporosis	Calcium, magnesium, boron, copper, sulfur
Arthritis	Calcium, magnesium, boron, copper, sulfur
Hypertension	Calcium, magnesium, boron
Bone spurs, heel spurs, calcium deposits	Calcium, magnesium, boron
Cancer	Selenium
Diabetes	Chromium, vanadium, zinc
Aneurysms	Copper
Cardiomyopathy	Selenium
Cataracts	Selenium
Deafness	Tin

OVEREATING AND BINGING

Another problem associated with malnourishment is **overeating** and **binging**. If you don't get the essential nutrients you need, your body will try to compensate, doing all it can to get more vitamins and minerals. In extreme cases, this phenomenon is known as **pica**, and it manifests itself as a craving for things commonly thought inedible. People with pica will lick dirt and chew wood; their bodies tell them to get the minerals they need in any way possible. In animals, pica is sometimes referred to as **cribbing**. It happens when farm animals gnaw on fences and metal bars. A farmer knows that when an animals cribs, it needs minerals![179]

Not all kinds of cravings for nutrients are quite as strange as pica and cribbing. More often, we simply go on binges to try to satisfy our need for vitamins and minerals. The sweet tooth you have might really be an urge for minerals; you eat and you eat but you never feel satisfied because you're lacking essential nutrients. For many people, malnourishment translates to over-eating and, eventually, obesity.

VITAMINS ARE VITAL TO YOUR DAILY LIFE

So far in this book, I've talked about **macronutrients**, which are the big food groups—proteins, sugar, and fats. Now, I'm going to discuss **micronutrients**, which are the small things your body needs to ingest: vitamins, minerals, and phytonutrients. Micronutrients don't produce energy on their own, but they play a role in turning macronutrients into energy.[180]

Vitamins are organic compounds required as nutrients in humans. Most scientists recognize 15 vitamins—five of which are part of the B complex—and we need all of them to stay alive. Vitamins can't be made in our bodies, so we have to get them from outside sources. Each vitamin does something different in our bodies, and each is essential. Read over the following table of essential vitamins to learn more about each one.[181]

ESSENTIAL VITAMINS

VITAMIN	DAILY VALUE (adults)	SOLUBILITY	FOOD SOURCES	DEFICIENCY SYMPTOMS	IMPORTANCE
A (beta carotene)	5,000 IU (international	Fat	Eggs, colored fruits and vegetables, dairy, fish liver oil	Teeth and gum problems, allergies, dry hair, eye irritations, sinus problems, night blindness	Healthy formation of bones, teeth and skin; tissue development, necessary for vision at night
B (complex)	See individual B vitamins	See individual B vitamins	Yeast, whole grains, liver	Dry skin, fatigue, constipation, acne, insomnia, lack of appetite	Nervous system function; skin and muscles; gives energy; boosts metabolism
B-1 (thiamin)	1.5 mg (milligrams)	Water	Nuts, wheat germ, fish, brown rice, whole wheat, legumes, organ meats	Constipation, depression, numbness of extremities, loss of appetite, noise sensitivity, impaired growth in children	Necessary in carbo metabolism; helps with digestion, growth, skin and eye health; essential for heart functioning
B-2 (riboflavin)	1.7 mg	Water	Dairy products, yeast, nuts, whole grains, molasses, organ meats	Poor digestion, inflammation of the mouth, eye problems, skin problems, dizziness	Helps with metabolism; necessary in making red blood cells; good for eyes, hair, nails, and skin
B-6 (pyridoxine)	2 mg	Water	Cabbage, cantaloupe, beans, peas, whole grains, yeast, leafy green vegetables	Loss of muscle control, insulin sensitivity, hair loss, irritability, learning disabilities, nervousness	Necessary for metabolism; helps with weight control; good for digestion, healthy skin, muscles, and nerves
B-12 (cobalamin)	6 mcg (micrograms)	Water	Dairy products, eggs, fish, beef, pork, organ meats	Tiredness, weakness, anemia, brain damage, nervousness, poor appetite	Necessary for red blood cell function; helps with metabolism, creates healthy cells and a healthy nervous system
Biotin (Vitamin H)	300 mcg	Water	Sardines, liver, egg yolks, beans, whole grains	Exhaustion, loss of appetite, impaired fat metabolism, depression, grayish skin, muscle pain	Helps with fatty acid production and growth promotion; boosts metabolism; good for skin, hair, and muscles
Choline	Not established	Water	Leafy green vegetables, egg yolks, fish, soybeans, organ meats	May lead to degeneration of liver, hemorrhaging of kidneys, intolerance to fats, ulcers, hypertension	May minimize fat in liver; helps with fat transport; regulates nerve transmission and gall bladder

ESSENTIAL VITAMINS (continued)

VITAMIN	DAILY VALUE (adults)	SOLUBILITY	FOOD SOURCES	DEFICIENCY SYMPTOMS	IMPORTANCE
Folic Acid (folate)	400 mcg	Water	Root vegetables, tuna, dairy products, leafy green vegetables, whole grains, oysters	Anemia, retarded growth, graying hair, gastrointestinal disorders	Necessary for cell growth and division, formation of red blood cells, and reproduction. Good for glands
Inositol	Not established	Water	Citrus, nuts, whole grains, vegetables, meat	Eye problems, skin problems, high cholesterol, constipation	Vital for hair growth and metabolism of fat; good for organs
B-5 (pantothenic acid)	10 mg	Water	Egg yolks, organ meats, yeast, beans, whole grains, mushrooms, salmon	Hypoglycemia, sensitivity to insulin, eczema, hair loss, stomach problems, kidney trouble	Resistance to stress; helps with energy; stimulates growth, helps form antibodies
Vitamin C (ascorbic acid)	60 mg	Water	Tomatoes, sprouts, citrus fruits, papaya, broccoli, strawberries, peppers	Weakness, anemia, skin hemorrhages, swollen joints, bleeding gums, low resistance to infections	Strengthens blood vessels, increased absorption of iron, resistance to infections; healthy teeth, gums, and bones
Vitamin D (calciferol))	400 IU	Fat	Fat, butter, fish oil, egg yolks, organ meat	May lead to rickets, lack of vigor, inadequate absorption of calcium, diarrhea, insomnia, soft bones, nervousness	Necessary for metabolism; helps with weight control; good for digestion, healthy skin, muscles, and nerves
Vitamin E (tocopherol)	30 IU	Fat	Cold pressed oils, whole wheat, sweet potatoes, nuts, dark vegetables, eggs, oatmeal, liver	Fragile red blood cells; dull hair; sterility and impotence; miscarriages; heart disease; gastrointestinal problems	Necessary for red blood cell function; helps with metabolism, creates healthy cells and a healthy nervous system
Vitamin K (bioflavinoi ds, rutin, hesperdin)	Not established	Fat	Cauliflower, fish oils, poly-unsaturated oils, eggs yolks, leafy greens	Hemorrhaging from prolonged clotting time; intestinal problems; miscarriages	Colds and flu prevention; healthy capillary walls; infrequent bruising

MINERALS MAKE YOUR BODY WORK

Minerals are simple, inorganic elements like calcium and potassium. Our bodies need more than 60 different minerals to survive! Of these 60, **16 essential minerals** are the most important. These are broken down into two groups—major minerals and minor minerals. The "major" group includes calcium, phosphorous, sodium, potassium, chloride, sulfur and magnesium; these seven elements are the most important minerals we need and should be ingested in daily doses of at least 100 mg. The remaining nine minerals are minor, which means our bodies' need them only in trace amounts. The minor minerals are: iron, selenium, copper, chromium, zinc, fluoride, manganese, molybdenum and iodine.

Like vitamins, minerals can't be synthesized within the body—we have to get them from outside sources, like food or supplements. But unlike vitamins, minerals aren't denatured during food preparation. With rare exceptions, minerals are just as effective after being heated as they are in raw food form. Still, it's nearly impossible to get all the

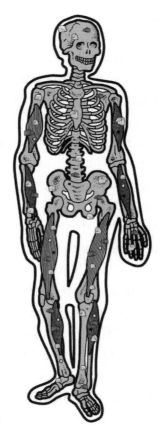

Vitamins & Minerals Make Your Body Work

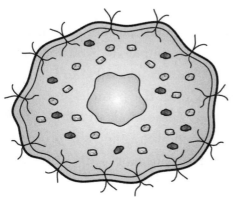

Vitamins & Minerals Make Cells Work

minerals you need from food alone. Supplementing is a must! However, not all mineral supplements are created equally.

THREE KINDS OF MINERALS

There are three different kinds of minerals available through supplements: **metallic, chelated,** and **colloidal. Metallic minerals** include those that are found in shells, limestone, mineral salt, sea water, and mineral oxides. They also turn up in clays, rocks, and antacids like Rolaids and Tums. In supplements, metallic minerals often take the form of tablets and powders called gluconate, lactate, sulfates, carbonates, and oxides.[182] They are only 8 to 12 percent biologically available to people younger than 40; people over 40 can only absorb about 3 to 5 percent of the mineral![183] Most of the minerals that you buy in a grocery store or pharmacy are metallic.

Chelated minerals are a bit better than their metallic counterparts. These forms of supplements, which were developed to nourish livestock, are created when an amino acid is wrapped around a mineral to make it more readily available. And it works. Approximately 40 percent of chelated mineral content can be absorbed by the body.

The best kinds of mineral supplements are **colloidal minerals,** which are from plants. The plants get minerals from the earth and make them into forms that are easily accessible to humans. Colloidal minerals are composed of ultra-fine particles suspended in a medium of a different matter. These kinds of supplements are incredibly bioavailable; 98 percent of the mineral is absorbed into the body![184] Colloidal mineral supplements are the products you should be looking for when you buy minerals.

Read over the following chart of essential minerals to learn more about the nutrients you should be supplementing.[185]

ESSENTIAL MINERALS

MINERAL	DAILY VALUE (adults)	DIETARY SOURCES	DEFICIENCY SYMPTOMS	IMPORTANCE
Calcium (Ca)	1000 mg	Leafy green vegetables, almonds, shellfish, dairy products	Back and leg pains, heart palpitations, tooth decay, muscle pains, brittle bones	Helps develop strong bones and teeth; assists with blood clotting, nerve transmission, heart rhythm
Chloride (Cl)	750 mg	Salt	Loss of muscle control, low blood pressure, weakness	Removes waste in the liver, regulates fluids, reduced acidity
Chromium (Cr)	120 mcg	Whole grains, clams, corn oil, yeast	Heart disease, intolerance in diabetes, depressed growth rate	Increases effectiveness of insulin; helps with metabolism; aids in synthesis of fatty acids and protein
Copper (Cu)	2 mg	Soybeans, raisins, nuts, fish, beans, organ meats	Skin sores, impaired breathing, weakness	Part of many enzymes; keeps skin healthy; helps form red blood cells
Fluoride (Fl)	10 mg	Tea, fish, tap water, foods cooked in tap water	Tooth decay	Helps with tooth enamel development and maintains bone structure
Iodine (I)	150 mcg	Mushrooms, fish, iodized salt	Obesity, irritability, cold hands and feet, dry hair, nervousness	Regulates rate of metabolism; enhances thyroid function; good for hair, nails, teeth, skin
Iron (Fe)	18 mg	Cherries, eggs, liver, fish, wheat, leafy green vegetables, dried fruit	Weakness, constipation, brittle bones, anemia	Needed to make red blood cells; promotes protein metabolism; helps resist stress and disease
Lithium (Li)	Not established	Foods grown in mineral-rich soil	Reduced fertility, depression, reduced longevity, slowed growth	Assists brain function; helps build strong muscles; regulates endocrine system
Magnesium (Mg)	400 mg	Whole grains, molasses, honey, nuts, green vegetables, fish	Confusion, tremors, nervousness	Good for energy; helps maintain bones, arteries, heart, nerves, and teeth
Manganese (Mn)	2 mg	Whole grains, nuts, beans, green vegetables, egg yolks, celery, pineapple	Hearing loss, dizziness, ataxia	Maintains sex hormone production; activates enzymes; needed for normal skeletal development
Molybdenum (Mo)	75 mcg	Beans, peas, lentils, grains	Very rare but leads to serious disease	Cofactor for a number of enzymes, helps with liver detoxification, breaks down waste products
Phosphorus (P)	1000 mg	Beans, dairy, nuts, eggs, fish, grains	Weight loss/gain, appetite loss, irregular breathing, fatigue, nervousness	Helps form bones and teeth; assists with cell growth and repair; contracts heart muscle
Potassium (K)	3500 mg	Whole grains, beans, dried fruits, peaches, nuts, seafood, bananas, apricots	Respiratory failure, cardiac arrest, poor reflexes, dry skin, irregular heartbeat, insomnia	Controls activity of heart muscles, nervous system, and kidneys; tranquilizes nerves
Selenium (Se)	70 mcg	Broccoli, onions, tuna, herring, whole grains	Premature aging	Works with Vitamin E; preserves tissue elasticity; helps proteins get utilized
Vanadium (V)	Not established	Shellfish, mushrooms, parsley, dill seed, black pepper	Depressed growth, impaired perinatal survival, enhanced levels of fats and plasma cholesterol	Regulates energy production; inhibits cholesterol synthesis; enhances bone and tooth formation
Zinc (Zn)	15 mg	Fish, soybeans, liver, spinach, mushrooms, sunflower seeds, organ meats	Sterility, delayed sexual maturity, loss of taste, poor appetite, fatigue	Component of insulin and semen; helps with burn and wound healing; aids in digestion and metabolism of protein.

COLORFUL PLATES ARE THE CHEAPEST INSURANCE POLICY

Have you ever heard of **phytonutrients**? These micronutrients are essential to health, but they're often overlooked. Phytonutrients

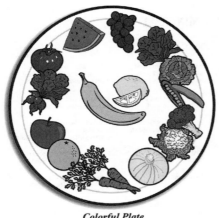

Colorful Plate

are biological substances that give fruits and vegetables their color, flavor, smell, and disease resistance.[186] They can play a huge role in preventing cancer and heart disease. Scientists estimate that there are as many as 40,000 phytonutrients in the world, but we only know of about 2,000.

It's easy to get a diverse variety of healthy phytonutrients into your diet: just make an effort to turn your dinner plate into a work of art. The more colors you eat, the better you're doing. Use the following table to learn about different phytonutrients and what they can do for your health.[187]

COLORFUL PHYTONUTRIENTS

COLOR	PHYTONUTRIENTS	SOURCE FOOD	DISEASE PROTECTION
Red	Lycopene	Tomatoes, guava, watermelon, red grapefruit	Heart disease, prostate cancer
Purple	Anthocyanidin, proanthocyanidin, resveratrol, flavinoids	Blueberries, blackberries, raspberries, grapes, red cabbage, red wine, eggplant, cranberry, pine bark, strawberries	Free radicals, arthritis, heart disease, premature aging, cancer
Yellow/ Green	Lutein, zeaxanthin	Spinach, kale, collards, curcumin, mustard greens, peas, romaine, soy	Blindness, vision problems
Green	Indoles, phenols, coumarins, isotheocyanates, dithiothiones, sulfuraphanes	Broccoli, cabbage, Brussels sprouts, kale, watercress, bok choy, collard greens	Cancer
White/ Green	Quercetin, polyphenols	Onions, garlic, green tea	Cancer, infection, viruses, liver toxins, cancels out free radicals
Orange	Cartenoids, especially beta-carotene	Carrots, cantaloupes, mangos, pumpkins, sweet potatoes, yams, apricots, squash	Cancer, heart disease, cancels out free radicals
Orange/ Yellow	Citrus bioflavinoids including rutin, quercetin, hesperidin, naringin	Lemons, limes, tangerines, oranges, other citrus fruit	Allergies, hemorrhaging, bruising, varicose veins, inflammation

FRACTAL NATURE OF FRUITS AND VEGETABLES

FRACTAL NATURE OF FRUITS AND VEGETABLES
God left us a clue as to what foods help what part of our body

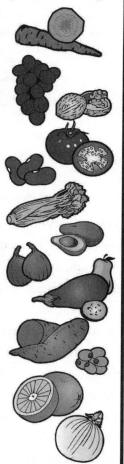

A sliced **carrot** looks like the human eye. Carrots greatly enhance blood flow to and function of the eyes.

Grapes hang in a cluster that has the shape of the heart. Each individual grape looks like a blood cell. Grapes are good for the heart.

A **walnut** looks like a little brain, a left and right hemisphere, upper cerebrums and lower cerebellums. Even the wrinkles or folds on the nut are just like the neo-cortex. Walnuts help brain function.

A **tomato** has four chambers and is red, just like our heart. Tomatoes are very beneficial for the heart.

Kidney beans actually heal and help maintain kidney function and yes, they look exactly like the human kidneys.

Celery, bok choy and rhubarb look just like bones and are 23% sodium - just like bones. These foods replenish the skeletal needs of the body.

Avocadoes target the health and function of the womb and cervix of the female - they look just like these organs. Avocadoes can balance hormones and prevent cervical cancers. And how profound is this? It takes exactly nine (9) months to grow an avocado from blossom to ripened fruit.

Figs are full of seeds and hang in twos when they grow. Figs increase the mobility of male sperm and increase the number of sperm as well to overcome male sterility.

Eggplant and pears also look just like the womb and cervix of the female and target the health and function of these organs.

Sweet potatoes are good for the pancreas and look just like one.

Olives assist the health and function of the ovaries.

Oranges, grapefruits, and other citrus fruits look just like the mammary glands of the female and actually assist the health of the breasts and the movement of lymph in and out of the breasts.

Onions look like the body's cells and help clear waste materials from all of the body cells. They even produce tears which wash the epithelial layers of the eyes.

STOP RUSTING!

What does a metal object do as it ages? It rusts! Your body does much the same thing. Rust is a form of oxidation, when electrons are taken away from atoms. Similarly, some cells in your body are

NATURAL ANTIOXIDANTS

ANTIOXIDANT	WHERE IT COMES FROM	WHAT IT DOES
Glutathione	Produced in the liver from three amino acids; can be gotten from fish, fresh fruits and vegetables, and meats. Milk thistle supplements may help your body make more of it.	Neutralizes free radicals produced from oxygen; detoxifies
SuperOxide Dismutase (SOD)	Made from copper, zinc, and manganese, which can be obtained through whole grains, nuts, egg yolks, and beans	Detoxifies superoxide, a free radical, into hydrogen peroxide. Then helps convert hydrogen peroxide to water
Catalase	Made in the body; can be increased with turmeric, green tea, bacopa, and milk thistle	Helps create smooth, younger looking skin; converts hydrogen peroxide to water.
Coenzyme Q10 (CoQ10)	Sardines, spinach, peanuts, beef, supplements	Helps produce energy; deficiencies associated with HIV, diabetes, heart disease, and periodontal disease
Lipolic Acid	Naturally occurring in most plants and animals. Can be synthesized by humans	Protects the liver and detoxifies the body after radiation and medication. Helps "recycle" other antioxidants; improves insulin metabolism.
Grape seed Extract	Grapes, red wine	Contains proanthocyanidins, antioxidants which are 20 times stronger than Vitamins C and E. Protects against vascular problems.

oxidized as you get older. The culprits behind this rust-like oxidation are **free radicals,** or molecules that are missing an electron. Free radicals "steal" electrons from other atoms, changing the atoms' chemical structure and causing problems along the way.[188]

Free radicals are produced in your body as a result of energy production. When substances are put together and broken down, molecules without electrons sometimes result. Excess free radicals can lead to cellular damage, which, when cumulative, can bring on cancer, heart disease, diabetes, and degenerative problems in the nervous system.[189]

To fight the effects of free radicals, give your body plenty of **antioxidants.** Antioxidants have an extra electron that they can donate to free radicals without harm. When free radicals get electrons from antioxidants, they don't wreak havoc on nearby cells. Out of the vitamins and minerals I've already mentioned, several are natural antioxidants, including **vitamins A, C,** and **E** and the minerals **selenium** and **zinc.** Foods rich in color that are packed with phytonutrients also tend to be good antioxidants.

Read over the previous chart to find out more about other kinds of antioxidants. And remember: it's best to get antioxidants from food rather than from supplements.[190]

NATURAL AND PROCESSED SUPPLEMENTS

I've already told you about processed minerals, which don't do much good because they can't be absorbed. Processed vitamins are also bad. These sometimes only include one component of the vitamin. The problem is that in nature, these vitamins are made up of multiple components. For example, many vitamin C supplements are made of only ascorbic acid. But in nature, the vitamin C complex contains ascorbic acid, copper, bioflavonoids, and many other factors, all of which make C much more effective.[191] Ascorbic acid on its own not only isn't effective, but it can also leach copper from your body to become more stable! It's a no-win situation when it comes to processed supplements.

Avoid buying **synthetic supplements** for the best health. A good rule of thumb is that if a supplement is sold in pharmacies or is made by pharmaceutical companies, it is most likely **overly processed**. This is not always the case, but the vast majority of commercially available supplements are bad for you. The cheapest products are generally not good; many cannot be absorbed into your body and contain harmful fillers that can be very toxic.[192] When it comes to your health, it's worth it to pay a little bit more to get a product that will do you good.

A very good way to find natural supplements is to visit an **herbologist**. An herbologist will recommend blends of herbs for you to take to eliminate toxins from your body.[193] He or she might provide you with tablet supplements, but your herbologist will also tell you about plants to eat that can provide you with nutrition. Herbal supplements can give all the vitamins and minerals you need for every organ system in your body. For example, regularly eating organic broccoli will provide you with just about every nutrient your body needs to stay healthy![194]

DON'T OVERDO IT!

Most things in large doses can make you sick. The same is true for some vitamins and minerals. **Fat-soluble vitamins,** like vitamins A, D, E and K, shouldn't be consumed in high doses. Unneeded fat-soluble vitamins are stored in fat deposits instead of being flushed out through the body; sometimes, too much of these vitamins can build up over time and lead to big problems. For example, too much vitamin A can cause liver disease. High doses of vitamin E can lead to heart disease.[195]

Some water-soluble vitamins can lead to bad side effects if they are consumed in very large doses too. For example, over-dosing on vitamin B_6 can lead to nerve damage in the arms and legs. And minerals should also be consumed in safe quantities. Too much selenium, for example, can lead to liver problems. To be safe, never take more than the recommended daily value of vitamins and minerals.[196]

TIMING IS EVERYTHING

Most things in the world follow patterns, including people. In fact, your body is on a 24-hour cycle called a **circadian rhythm.** Because of this natural rhythm, your body functions differently at different times of the day. Sometimes, you're naturally active, but other times, you might feel like you've been drained of all your energy.

You have to respect your body's cycle when taking your supplements. When the proper supplements are taken at appropriate times, they are most effective. The idea that supplements are best used at different times of the day is called **chrononutrition**. "Chrono" means time, so chrononutrition is simply the study of how time affects the body's benefit from vitamins, minerals, herbs, and other dietary supplements. Following the principles of chrononutrition, your supplements should be divided into three packets: some for morning, some for afternoon, and some to take just before bed. I will talk more about chrononutrition in the metabolism section of this book.

CAN YOU DIGEST ALL OF THIS?

Vitamins, minerals, phytonutrients, antioxidants . . . there's a lot of stuff that needs to go into your body! So far, you've realized that you have to take supplements of essential nutrients and eat colorful foods to stay healthy. But all of these nutrients won't help if you can't break them down through digestion. Therefore, more supplements are required—**hydrochloric acid** and **digestive enzymes**. Specifically, you need to make sure your body has the pancreatic enzymes necessary for splitting apart foods: lipase, protease, and amylase.[197]

Probiotics are also important to digestive health, and they can be found in fermented foods like sauerkraut, soy sauce, Kimchi, and organic yogurt. Probiotics are "friendly" bacteria that live in your intestines. They help you break down and absorb the food you eat. You have more than 100 trillion bacteria in your intestines alone, and it's important that you have plenty of good strains available to properly balance your system.[198] A strong army of friendly bacteria can contribute to your health by strengthening your immune system, helping with digestion, removing toxins from your system, and even creating B vitamins.[199]

You should always try to supplement probiotics, but getting

good bacteria into your body is especially important when you are stressed, have had antibiotic treatments, are on estrogen, or have done lots of traveling. In these situations, your body's balance of bacteria may be off kilter, so regular supplements are needed.[200] Also, anyone over the age of 50 should supplement probiotics regularly. Although there are hundreds of strains of good probiotics, *Lactobacillus acidophilus* and *Bifidobacterium* are the most common kinds available. Try to supplement with at least 10 billion living cells of these strains daily.[201] Most probiotic supplement products meet this requirement.

EXERCISE: ADDING SUPPLEMENTS TO YOUR LIFE

Write down all the vitamins and minerals you take now:

If necessary, decide which additional supplements you'll take daily:

When will you take these supplements?

WHAT IS SALT?

Salt is essential to all life on earth.[202] It is one of the most important ingredients for life, and all living things utilize it.[203] Salt is also the **spice of life**—it makes food taste better.[204] Chemically, simple salt is a compound produced when sodium (Na+), a metal so unstable that is easily bursts into flame, combines with chlorine (Cl-), a deadly poisonous gas. When they come together and stabilize, they are neither explosive nor poisonous.[205]

A healthy adult's body contains about 250 grams of salt, which would fill three large salt shakers.[206] Salt is found on the ground in dry salt beds, in the oceans, in underground springs, and in rocks under the earth.[207] The ocean is the most common area to harvest salt for consumption. However, it takes more than a year to naturally produce sea salt with the help of the wind and the sun![208]

HISTORY OF SALT

Salt was once thought to be very rare. People treasured it. They traded for salt. They built roads just to transport salt. They fought wars over salt. They even used salt for money.[209] Salt was even revered in language; the words "salary," "salad," "soldier," "salami," "sausage," and "sauce" all were derived from salt.[210]

Before the advent of the refrigerator, salt was used to **preserve food** by killing bacteria and drawing off moisture. Milk and cream were cured with salt to become cheese. Cabbage was cured to make sauerkraut; cucumbers to pickles; pork to ham or bacon.[211] Over the years, salt has been used for making paper, plastics, PVC, glass, antifreeze, laundry detergent, soft drinks, pharmaceuticals, new explosives, and many other products.[212] [213]

FUNCTIONS OF SALT

According to the National Academy of Sciences, the average adult needs 2300 mg of salt daily. That is equivalent to about **one teaspoon of salt**.[214] Without the adequate amount of salt, nothing will work in your body. You won't be able to think or move at all. Salt is needed for breathing, digestion, nutrient transport, oxygen dispersal, and nerve impulses.[215] Salt also combines with potassium to regulate the acid-alkaline balance in your blood and help control your heart beat.[216] It is necessary for your metabolism to function, to promote detoxification, and for optimization of your hormonal, nervous, and immune systems.[217] Salt even regulates the movement of water in and out of the cells through the process of **osmosis,** which controls all of your metabolic functions.

Salt is wonderful for the outside of your body too. Extremely salty water can help relieve many skin problems. For example, the Dead Sea is 10 times saltier than the ocean, and Utah's Great Salt Lake is six times saltier than the ocean.[218] [219] When you soak your body in these places, skin ailments like eczema and psoriasis will improve and sore muscles will be alleviated. Soaking in highly concentrated salt water will be relaxing, energizing, and rejuvenating too.[220]

WHITE GOLD TO WHITE POISON

Salt used to be called **"white gold"** because it was so precious and natural. In recent years, however, salt has turned into **"white poison."** It is now regularly **processed** to lengthen its shelf life and improve its appearance. Chemicals such as sulfuric acid and chlorine are used to remove minerals in natural salt. Then, high pressure and heat are used to evaporate water in the salt. This refining process disrupts the compound's molecular structure and devitalizes salt. In addition, anti-caking agents such as sodium ferrocyanide, ammonium citrate, and aluminum silicate are used to prevent this refined salt from sticking together.[221] These additives make the salt even more toxic!

In the 1920s, iodide was first added to **refined salt** to prevent goiter, a hypothyroid condition caused by lack of iodine in the diet. Iodizing salt was meant to stop epidemic spread of goiter, but it is not extremely effective. That's because only 10 percent of the iodide added to iodized salt is available for absorption.[222] Fluoride is also added to refined salt, supposedly to strengthen our teeth. However, both the iodine and fluoride components are aggressive and harmful.[223] The final salt product is lifeless, devoid of any healthful minerals. It is 99.7 to 99.95 percent plain sodium chloride.

Unrefined natural salt, on the other hand, is harvested without any processing. Salt collectors use only wind and sun to dry the salt.[224] This process takes over a year. The final product contains more than 80 minerals, including sulfur, magnesium, potassium, calcium, silicon, iron, and many others. The best natural salts available are **Redmond Real Salt®** from Utah, **Celtic Sea Salt®** from France, and **Himalayan Crystal Salt** from the Himalayan Mountains.

PROCESSED SALT EPIDEMIC

I truly believe that our consumption of refined, processed salt is one of the **biggest health problems** we face in the world right now. When refined salt is used for everything in our food supply, it creates havoc in our systems. Since salt is the most important element for transportation of fluids in our bodies, processed salt causes a total imbalance across the board. When we have too much refined salt without other minerals to balance it out, water quickly moves from the inside of cells to the outside through osmosis. This dehydrates the cell, causes chronic diseases such as cancer, and eventually leads to cell death. When we have unrefined natural salt with a plethora of minerals in our extra-cellular and intracellular fluid, water will not move out of cells to dehydrate them. You really need to supplement unrefined natural salt daily to ensure a perfect balance for your cellular system.[225]

A LOW SALT DIET IS DANGEROUS

Two of the biggest health myths of all time are about salt. These myths are that salt is bad for you and that it causes hypertension. Both are **not true!** Only refined salt is bad. In fact, many studies prove that a low-salt diet actually increases hypertension.[226] In 1984, the National Health and Nutritional Examination Survey (NHANES) revealed that a pattern of low mineral intake, specifically magnesium, potassium and calcium was directly associated with hypertension. Over the past 20 years, repeated measurements have confirmed the relationship between low mineral intake and elevated blood pressure.

Refined artificial salt primarily contains sodium and chloride. Unrefined natural salt has a wide range of minerals including potassium and magnesium. Magnesium is nature's relaxation mineral. It relaxes the smooth muscles of the blood vessels to decrease blood pressure. Potassium from the natural salt moves into the cells and draws extra-cellular fluid out. This lowers the blood volume outside of cells hence the blood pressure. This is the process that occurs when natural salt lowers blood pressure.

In addition, a low-salt diet causes higher total cholesterol and lousy LDL cholesterol levels.[227] It also increases adrenal hormones such as aldosterone, rennin, angiotensinm, and nora-drenaline to cause heart attacks. Insulin levels are increased with refined salt as well, bringing about diabetes, obesity, and polycystic ovary syndrome.[228]

When you lack unrefined salt, you can accumulate too many toxic elements in your system, leading to delirium, psychomotor retardation, schizophrenia, and hallucinations.[229] Toxic elements are everywhere, and without natural salt to regulate them, they build up in your body. For example, bromide is in many substances such as antibacterial agents for pools and hot tubs, fumigants for agriculture, pest and termite products, fire retardants, carbonated drinks such as Mountain Dew®, energy drinks, Gatorade®, bakery products such as breads, cookies, cakes, and many prescription medications.[230]

Additionally, in order for your thyroid hormones to function optimally, inactive T4 hormones need to be converted to active T3 hormones. When you are deficient in minerals and have adrenal exhaustion, T4 will not convert to T3 form. Unrefined salt provides the proper balance of minerals to ensure proper thyroid functions.[231] It helps all your hormone systems work properly.

SALT THERAPY

Our blood is a 1 percent salt solution, which is equal to the salt concentration of the oceans.[232] When you keep your insides well balanced with unrefined salt, you will be able to attain great health. I believe everyone will benefit from my salt therapy regimen. It entails ingesting **unrefined natural salt** daily, a **monthly salt bath** or **daily foot soaks, upper respiratory cleansing,** and installing **salt lamps** inside the home. More details about my salt regimen are described below:

UNREFINED SALT needs to be ingested daily. For every quart of water you drink, you should have ¼ tablespoon of unrefined salt.[233] So I usually recommend that my patients to take **one teaspoon** of unrefined salt first thing in the morning when they wake up. Some people can't tolerate this at first, so I have them start with a pinch and work up to one teaspoon. The dose is very salty and difficult to ingest for me too, so I take encapsulated unrefined salt. In pill form, you can't taste the saltiness.

TAKING A SALT BATH is a powerful way to detoxify. In fact, 30 minutes of a salt bath is equivalent to **three days of fasting,** in terms of detoxification. Minerals from the salt are absorbed through the skin, and toxins are released into the bath water through osmosis. The most effective time to bathe with salt is during a full moon. The powerful tide of the moon enhances the whole detoxification process.

To create your bath, put one to two pounds of crystal salt in your bathtub. Then, add just enough water to cover the salt for 30 minutes. After the half hour is up, fill the tub the rest of the way. Maintain the temperature of the water near your body temperature of 98.6 degrees Fahrenheit at all times. Soak for 15 to 30 minutes. When you're done with your bath, don't shower; simply pat yourself dry with a towel. Rest for at least 30 minutes after you enjoy your salt soak.[234]

If you'd prefer, you can soak your feet daily instead of taking a full bath. Add 2 tablespoons of natural salt for each quart of warm water. Soak your feet for 15 minutes. This will help eliminate athlete's foot in one month and fungal nails in about 3 months. I am currently conducting a clinical trial using salt therapy for fungal nail condition with seminar participants. For the past 18 years, I have been extremely frustrated with the lack of improvement of fungal nail conditions using current medical treatments. Soaking should also help warts and insect bites as well.

UPPER RESPIRATORY SALT CLEANSING is an extremely effective way to fight upper respiratory diseases such as the flu, sinus infection, hay fever, sore throat, runny nose, allergic eye infection, bronchitis and asthma. Since so many people suffer from flu every year, and flu vaccinations are toxic and ineffective in many cases, I recommend sinus flushes during the flu season to combat and prevent the flu.

For **sinus flush,** use one half cup of warm water and add one half teaspoon of natural salt. Tilt your head back. Use your right thumb to close your right nostril and pour a small amount of the salt water slowly into your left nostril. Suck it into your left nostril and spit out through your mouth. Reverse this process for your other nostril. Repeat this process several times in each nostril. Repeat this one to two times a day. You might want to use an eye dropper to make it easier to insert the water. This process will eliminate any symptoms of the flu and may prevent you from getting the flu. Try this when you travel and are not able to rest.

For **sore throat**, gargle with warm salt water daily. I also recommend using eye wash daily during the flu season or when you have eye infection. You can use an eye wash cup or small shot glass to wash your eyes. For more serious conditions such as bronchitis and asthma, I recommend salt inhalation treatment. Bring salt water to a boil, cool until you can inhale the fumes without burning your nostrils. Do this treatment daily for 10 to 15 minutes.

SALT LAMPS are powerful ways to detoxify the inside of your homes. You should do all you can to cleanse your home's interior. Average Americans spend 65 to 90 percent of their lives indoors, and inside environments are five times more polluted than outdoor ones![235] Salt lamps emit negatively charged ions to decrease indoor pollutants such as bacteria, fungi, pollen, dust mites, animal dander, and mold. They are natural **air purifiers and ionizers**[236] that don't require a large investment or costly filter replacements.

TVs and computers produce an electromagnetic frequency of around 100 to 160 hertz. Our brain waves vibrate at around 8 hertz. That means our bodies are regularly exposed to frequencies that vibrate 20 times faster than our brains! This can lead to a lack of concentration, nervousness, insomnia, and cancer. Salt lamps' negatively charged ions bind to excessive positive ions to neutralize these **electromagnetic pollutions**. When the light is turned on, it travels through the salt to create positive energy and attract humidity to act as a **natural humidifier**.[237]

There will be more information on salt therapy in my

upcoming book, *9 Secrets of Salt—Unlocking the Healing Power of Natural Salt*. In this book, we will go beyond the physical benefits of salt, exploring the emotional and spiritual aspects inherent in becoming the salt of the earth.

SCHEDULE YOUR HEALTH

You need to take supplements three times each day—some in the morning with breakfast, some with lunch, and some in the evening with dinner. When do you supplement? Draw your answer in the blank chart below.

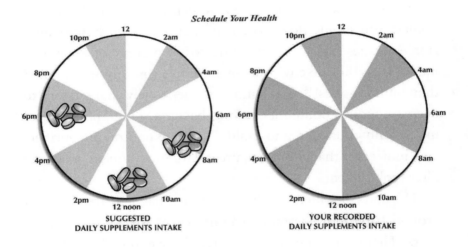

Schedule Your Health

SUGGESTED
DAILY SUPPLEMENTS INTAKE

YOUR RECORDED
DAILY SUPPLEMENTS INTAKE

METAL WELLNESS SCORING CHART

This chart is simple. Give yourself is a point if you more of your circles are above the dotted line. If more circles are on the bottom, you don't get any points.

Vitamins & Minerals Wellness Scoring Chart
Circle what you eat

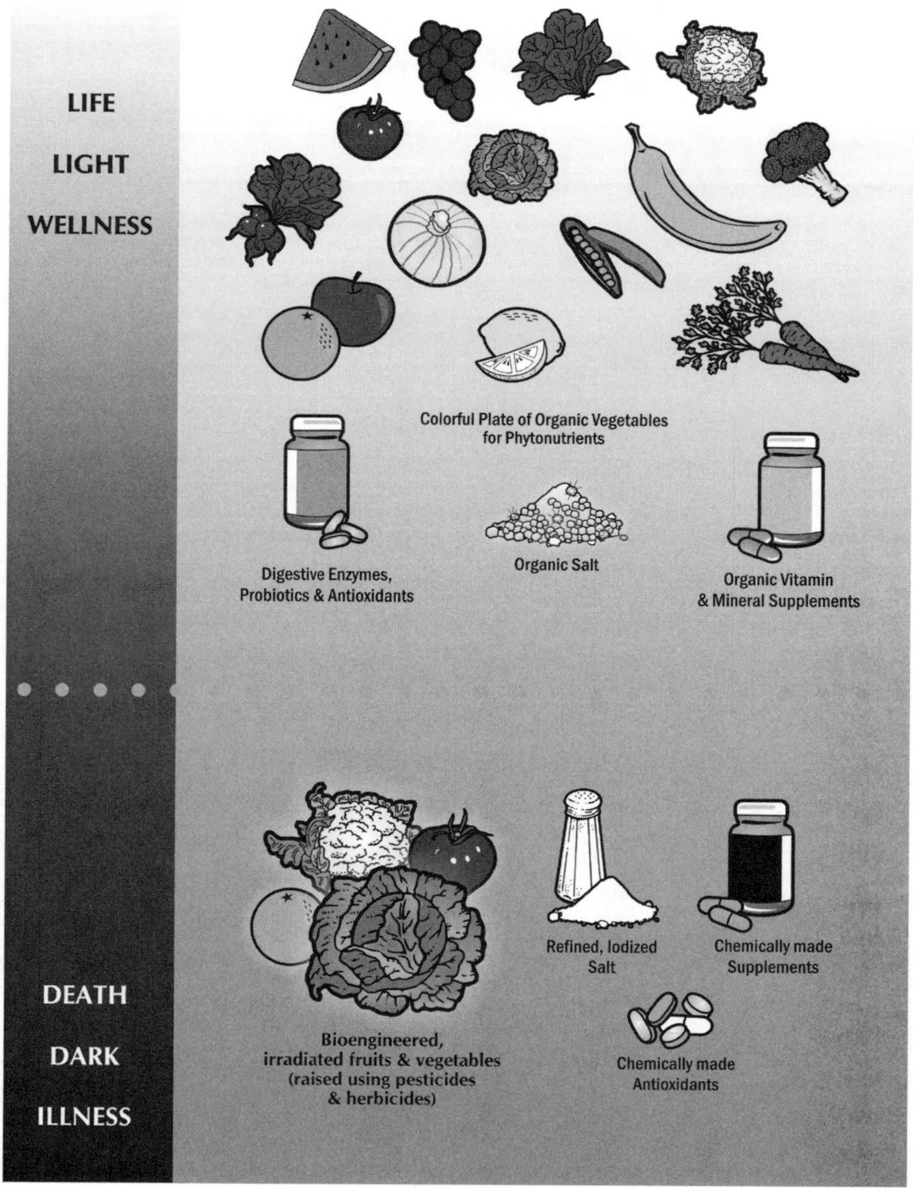

LIFE

LIGHT

WELLNESS

Colorful Plate of Organic Vegetables
for Phytonutrients

Digestive Enzymes,
Probiotics & Antioxidants

Organic Salt

Organic Vitamin
& Mineral Supplements

DEATH

DARK

ILLNESS

Bioengineered,
irradiated fruits & vegetables
(raised using pesticides
& herbicides)

Refined, Iodized
Salt

Chemically made
Supplements

Chemically made
Antioxidants

Chapter 7

THE 6TH SECRET:
WIND

"EXERCISE AND WALK"

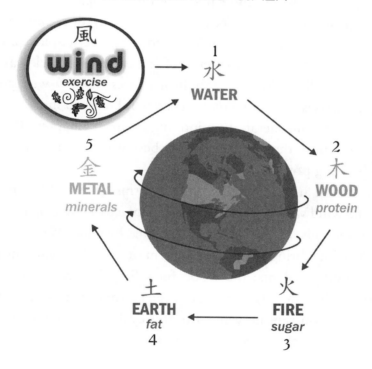

When the wind blows, the earth rotates. Along the same lines, breathing and exercise creates movement in our bodies, which makes our metabolisms work properly. Lack of movement or exercise causes stagnant energy that is toxic to our bodies. Walking is by far the easiest and healthiest exercise. When you walk

10,000 steps a day, you will be physically, mentally and spiritually healthy. I will introduce my nine wellness dowel exercises later on in this chapter to promote stretching, strengthening, breathing, and balance all at once.

THE WIND HAS TO BLOW

So far, you've learned about the five elements of earth and how they translate into your own life. But the fact is that you can drink plenty of water and eat all the right things and still have health problems. That's because if your body does not move and breathe, you are in trouble. Wind, or exercise, plays a big role in moving the five elements of the earth in a cycle called your **metabolism**. Your metabolism relates to how well your body processes food and creates energy. I'll tell you more about how to turn your metabolism into high gear in Chapter 10, but for now, know that exercise is the best way to amp up your metabolizing power.

Let's look at the title illustration for this chapter. I'll explain how the wind works. The five elements of earth make up a cycle that never ends, and this cycle is mediated by wind. Wind blows clouds, which brings water in the form of rain. The water nourishes wood or plants; the wood fuels fire; the fire burns into ash or earth; minerals come out of the earth; minerals melt into water. The constant movement of this cycle is created by wind, which is the sixth secret of my nine secrets to health.

YOU ARE NOT MOVING ENOUGH

Unfortunately, most Americans aren't exercising enough. Studies show that only 22 percent of American adults get enough exercise during their leisure time to receive health benefits.[238] And many people suffer because of their **lack of exercise**. Insomnia, for example, can usually be attributed to insufficient movement. People aren't able to sleep because their bodies aren't tired. They don't use enough energy all day, so their bodies don't think they need to rest.[239]

The sedentary problem started about 100 years ago, when **cars** began to be mass produced. People no longer had to walk to get around; they could drive. It got even worse after **TV** became popular in the 1950s. **Remote**-controlled television further exacerbated the situation. With the advent of the remote, people no longer even had to get up to change the channel! Now, with **computers** filling workplaces and **video games** becoming the norm in every household, people have even more reasons to keep from being active. Exercising has become something that we don't do automatically; nowadays, we have to plan for it. Some people say they don't have time for working out, but that excuse doesn't hold water for most Americans. A 2003 poll found that the average American adult has 5.1 hours of free time each day. Sadly, the majority of people spend over half that time watching TV.

In my own experience, when I tell people to exercise, many people claim that they are too tired to do anything after a day at work. However, exercising is a good way to perk up. I know that when I come home after a long day of seeing patients, I am dead tired until I exercise. But after a good workout, I feel energized. You get more energy when you exercise, so using the "too tired" excuse really isn't valid.

YOU ARE PARKED TOO LONG AND TOO WRONG

Sitting down might be conducive to working, but it's not good for your health. As the illustrations below show, parking your

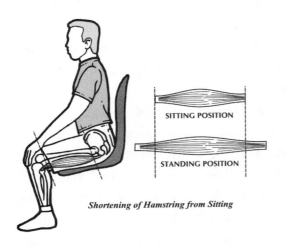

SITTING POSITION

STANDING POSITION

Shortening of Hamstring from Sitting

body in a seated position creates **tight hamstrings** and out-of-whack **hip muscles**, which can cause your pelvis to move out of place. In fact, most people who sit all day have either an **anterior or posterior pelvic tilt.** An anterior pelvic tilt is when the pelvis points downward due to weak hamstrings and stronger thighs and hip flexors. A posterior pelvic tilt, on the other hand, happens when the pelvis points upwards; it's caused by tight hip flexors and abdominal muscles.[240] Both kinds of pelvis problems happen when people sit all day, moving their upper bodies but ignoring their lower halves. This isn't good. Tilted pelvises equal **poor posture.** And eventually, a tilted pelvis can cause back pain.[241]

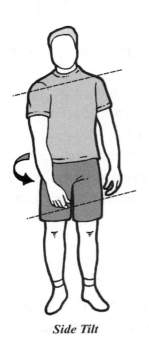

Side Tilt

You can also develop postural problems when you **favor one side of your body** over the other. This is common in athletes who play sports that require the use of only one hand. If you favor one arm over the other when carrying bags or lifting, you might develop postural problems as well. Favoring one side over the other causes one side of your body to be higher; your hip and shoulder on

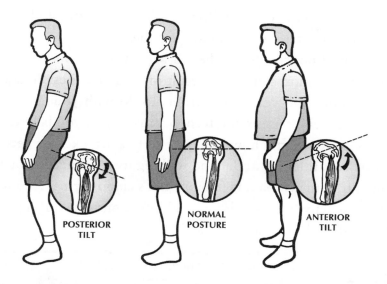

POSTERIOR
TILT

NORMAL
POSTURE

ANTERIOR
TILT

one half will literally be raised above the other side, making you uneven.[242]

I see postural problems everyday in my practice. These imbalances in the back and hips cause the majority of foot, ankle, knee, hip, low back, and neck problems. And many of the postural problems are rooted in inactivity. In other words, sitting too long and favoring one side is hurting your body. All of your musculoskeletal problems could be traced back to these habits!

WHY DO YOU HAVE TO EXERCISE?

When you park your body in a chair all day, your skeleton gets all out of whack. But you also experience other negative consequences beyond structural problems. Your brain suffers, your muscles deteriorate, and almost everything inside of you stops functioning to its fullest potential. The health problems associated with a sedentary lifestyle are devastating!

When you do exercise, on the other hand, you reap the

rewards. Look over the following chart to learn all about the good things exercise can do for your health.[243]

A lot of positive bodily health benefits come out of exercising, but the most important result of an active lifestyle doesn't have to do with your body. It has to do with your mind and spirit. Exercise raises **self esteem** because it gets you believing in yourself. No matter how little you do to start, exercise gets you away from thinking about and wishing for a change in your life and into actually making it happen. It's **empowering**! And when physical activity joins with mental **intentions**—having a goal in mind—health benefits increase.[244]

EXERCISE DOES GREAT THINGS FOR YOUR HEALTH!	
EXERCISE INCREASES...	EXERCISE DECREASES...
Lung capacity, lymphatic flow for toxin elimination, digestive effectiveness, bone strength, energy, metabolism, ability to sleep, sweat levels for detoxification	Stress, memory loss, risk of Alzheimer's disease, risk of Parkinson's disease, depression, weight, likelihood of cancer, diabetes, and heart attack, effects of aging; pain, susceptibility to cold and flu

YOU NEED LOTS OF OXYGEN

I like to call oxygen "vitamin O" because you depend on it so much. You can live up to six weeks without food. You can live up to a week without water. But after two minutes without oxygen, you're dead. As you can see in the pictures, oxygen circulates throughout your body and into each of your cells. Every part of you needs oxygen to stay alive. It's the most important thing you put into your body by far.

Unfortunately for us humans alive today, we don't have access to as much oxygen as our early ancestors. Our atmospheric oxygen levels have dropped significantly in the last few thousand years; now only 21 percent of the air is oxygen![245] To take advantage of the most oxygen you can, you need to breathe deeply and get your lungs in shape. And the best way to condition your lungs is to do aerobic exercise. As its name implies, **aerobic exercise** uses air—oxygen—to get work done. This kind of exercise uses large muscle groups in a rhythmic, uninterrupted, submaximal fashion.[246] Examples of aerobic exercise include anything that gets your heart pumping: running, walking, skating, cross-country skiing, rope jumping, stair climbing, rowing, and swimming. All aerobic exercises help your body provide oxygen to your musculoskeletal system more effectively.[247] In other words, aerobic exercises improve your cardiovascular system so that it can help your muscles work better.

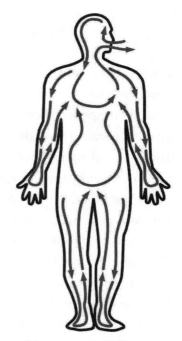

Movement of Oxygen in Your Body

The source of energy in cardiovascular exercise is fat; when you get your heart rate up and you start breathing heavy, the energy from fat is what keeps you going. Regular aerobic exercise, therefore, can help you lose weight; it can also increase your basal metabolic rate, or BMR, which measures how many calories your body uses each day. Your lung capacity will also

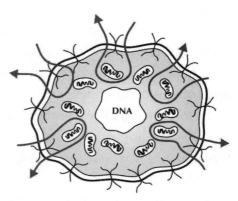

Movement of Cell with Oxygen

increase over time with aerobic exercise, and when your lungs have expanded, you'll be much less likely to catch a cold.

YOU NEED MORE MUSCLES

I have many senior patients come to see me in my practice. It upsets me to see that many of them can't get off the exam table after their appointments. Their inability to move isn't due to old age; it's because they don't have enough **muscle strength**. This is always a sad sight to see because I know such problems could be prevented with strength training. Research shows that we lose 10 ounces of muscle every year after the age of 40. That's the equivalent of a medium-sized steak! Another study shows that we lose 1 percent in muscle mass every year after the age of 50.[248] If you do nothing, you'll be like my senior patients after a while, too weak to lift your own body. There's only one way to fight muscle loss—with anaerobic exercise, or **strength training.**

Think about these amazing numbers: there are 639 muscles in your body, and each one has about 10 million muscle cells. That means you have about 6 billion muscle cells total, all of which help you move.[249]**Anaerobic exercise** is the only way to increase and maintain this muscle mass safely. Strength training also increases your metabolism, reduces body fat, increases bone density, helps with digestion, helps lower blood pressure and cholesterol, reduces arthritis pain, eases low back pain, and gives you extra confidence.[250]

Beyond being the power behind your every movement, muscles are also important because they **store water and sugar** for future use. Their amazing storage potential explains why you are dehydrated and crave sugar when you don't have developed muscles; your body can't hold all the water and sugar it could with muscle mass! They also determine where your bones go in your body, holding your skeleton in the right place. Without muscles, your bones would collapse on the floor. And since muscles play a big role in the placement of your bones, they also hugely influence your posture.[251]

BACK EQUALS TO FOOT

Your foot is representative of your whole body—it's another example of the fractal geometry I mentioned in Chapter One. Chinese medicine has known this for thousands of years. In Chinese medicine, treating a part of the foot can help heal other parts of the body too.

As you can see in the following illustration, the ball of your foot coincides with your upper back, and the heel with your tailbone. Therefore, the arch of your foot is in line with your spine. These areas in both the foot and the spine are formed around ball-and-socket joints. When the arch of your foot collapses, your spine will bend forward and the back will flatten. Similarly, when your arches are too high, your spine is overly

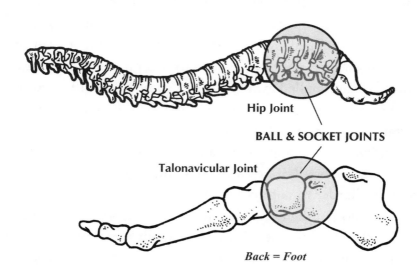

Hip Joint

BALL & SOCKET JOINTS

Talonavicular Joint

Back = Foot

arched too. As a foot and ankle specialist, my primary job is to get people back on their feet without pain. Because of the connection between feet and backs, most of my patients with foot ailments also have back issues. I always support their feet to stabilize the foundation of their bodies. But I also teach them back strengthening exercises to make sure that they are covered on both ends of the body. When their backs get better, their foot condition improves and vice versa.

SPINE HEALTH

Your back is very delicate. The individual bones in your spine are held together by gel, called discs. Since there's only gel holding together your spine, the integrity of your back depends on conditioning your **back muscles**. With strong back muscles, your back will be better able to develop good posture. Underdeveloped back muscles, however, are a recipe for disaster.

It's crucial that you exercise your back to develop your muscles. Unfortunately, our lifestyles nowadays make getting our backs into shape harder than it would have been in the past. These days, most of us spend the vast majority of working hours slumped over a computer. Our shoulders fall forward in a seated position, leading to bad posture. Ideally, they would remain pulled away from our chests. But with forward-facing shoulders, our rib cages close in on themselves, and our organs are put in precarious positions. What's more, as we get older, our shoulders naturally bow forward, regardless of whether you sit all day or not. So if you're over 50, you'll have to work harder to correct your posture.

How do you fight back against the poor posture generated by a sedentary lifestyle? With exercise. I've developed an easy strengthening exercise system for you to follow. It's listed at the end of this chapter. With my system, you'll develop the "wings" of your back—your upper back muscles surrounding your shoulder blades—which will help you open up your chest, square your shoulders, and straighten out your neck and back muscles. If you do my dowel exercises each day, you'll straighten out your back and protect your spine.

"WALKING IS MAN'S BEST MEDICINE." -HIPPOCRATES

Hippocrates, who is considered to be the father of modern medicine, treated many illnesses with morning and evening walks.[252] He recognized the value that walking has for human health and human spirits. **Walking** is an easy aerobic exercise; it's safe, inexpensive, convenient, suitable for all levels, and requires no training or equipment.[253] There are unbelievable benefits to walking. Not only can a nightly stroll increase your **cardiovascular health** and refine your **musculoskeletal system,** but it can also improve your **mental performance** and your **self esteem.** Walking provides all the benefits of more intensive cardiovascular exercise without the high impact level. It leads to better breathing, a stronger heart, lower blood pressure, lower cholesterol, stronger immunity, increased muscular strength, improved balance and flexibility, stronger bones, better sleep, and less depression.[254]

The rhythmic movement of walking synchronizes your brain waves to relieve anxiety.[255] It also boosts your imagination, sometimes being the perfect catalyst for a good idea. [256] Walking increases productivity and makes creative breakthroughs more likely.[257] It's an excellent way to interact with nature. Walking also gives you time alone, which you can spend thinking about renewal and realignment.[258] When you walk, you will fully understand the amazing design of your body. As you can see, there's a whole lot more to walking than just moving your feet.

10,000 STEPS A DAY

Walking is an activity that most people do everyday. You walk around your house, you walk to your car, and you walk around your office at work. But for the majority of Americans, daily walking is limited to the bare minimum. Most people take between 2,000 and 4,000 steps each day.[259] That seems like a lot, but in actuality we need to take about **10,000 steps** each day to stay healthy.[260] And if you want to lose weight, the number of steps you should take increases to between 12,000 and 15,000.[261] You have to make an effort to take that many steps. Buy a simple pedometer to measure your steps and see how many you take now. What do you have to do to increase your daily steps to a healthy level?

Once you've committed to walking more, all you have to do is get up and go! But before you start any aerobic walk, you need to **warm up** and **stretch** for about five minutes.[262] Be careful not to overstretch before walking. If you stretch too much before your muscles get warm, you could easily hurt yourself.[263] Once you start walking, try to keep your breathing regular. Breathe in for three counts and out for three counts to make sure you're taking deep, oxygen-filled breaths. Deep breathing gives your body plenty of life-giving oxygen, and it also calms the mind and relaxes your muscles.

When you first start to walk, you may not be able to go very far. That's okay. It's good enough that you're getting up and moving. Set a goal for yourself in distance, steps, or time walked. Then, work toward that goal, increasing your walk by a few minutes each day. Repeating an affirmation can help make your walk a more positive experience by making you aware of your choice to get healthy.[264] Chant a powerful expression like "**I am fit, I am healthy**" or "**I can do it**" to keep you motivated.

INSTEAD OF WALKING

Almost everyone can walk for fitness, but I don't recommend it for people who are extremely overweight. In fact, I don't recommend any weight-bearing exercise for overweight people. Weight-bearing activities, like walking, running, or jumping, can put undue pressure on the joints in overweight people, causing damage. Therefore, I recommend **cycling** or **swimming** for anyone who is seriously overweight. After you get close to your ideal weight, you can take up walking if you wish. However, continuing with swimming or biking is fine too.

You can opt to swim or bike even if you are at a healthy weight. Some people don't like walking for one reason or another; don't feel that you have to do it if it's something you don't enjoy. Just do some sort of exercise to substitute. If you decide to swim or bike, know that you can convert swimming or cycling workouts to steps to get an idea of how much you would be walking. Simply give yourself 110 steps for every minute you spend swimming or biking.[265] You can use the chart below as a reference.[266]

STEP CONVERSION CHART	
MINUTES CYCLING or SWIMMING	**STEPS EARNED**
15	1,650
20	2,200
30	3,300
45	4,950
60	6,600
90	9,900

MORE WALKING

In my Nine Week Life Transformation Program, I have the participants increase their walking steps by 10 to 20 percent each week. Doing this can be a good way to add structure to your workout. Follow the next chart to find out how many steps to add each week. This chart increases by 20 percent each week. You can start with as many steps as you feel are right for you.

WEEKLY STEPS WALKED					
WEEK	**STEPS (select your number of steps to start with and continue down that column)**				
1	1000	2000	3000	4000	5000
2	1200	2400	3600	4800	6000
3	1400	2800	4300	5800	7200
4	1700	3500	5200	7000	8600
5	2000	4000	6200	8300	10,000
6	2500	5000	7500	10,000	12,000
7	3000	6000	9000	12,000	14,000
8	3600	7000	10,000	14,000	17,000
9	4500	8500	12,000	17,000	20,000

If you want more bang for your buck on your walk, try using my wellness dowel. The dowel is useful in my strengthening exercises, which I will describe further on. But it can also help on an aerobic walk. The dowel disassembles to become two walking sticks. If you hold these sticks in your hands with your arms bent at a 90-degree angle, you'll burn more calories and tone your upper body along the way.[267]

MANY WALKS OF LIFE

To make things easier, I've identified styles of walking based on steps per minute. A stroll is approximately 60 steps per minute. In a **stroll**, you walk at a leisurely pace and don't feel tired after a long time. The next step up in walking intensity doubles the number of steps per minute; I call this walk a **health walk**. At 120 steps per minute, a health walk should be easy to maintain but tiring after a while. On a health walk, you should be able to carry on a conversation with a friend. Talking during a **weight-loss walk,** however, might be uncomfortable. The pace on this kind of walk is 135 steps each minute. Finally, an **aerobic walk** packs in 150 steps per minute. On an aerobic walk, you'll have trouble breathing; you won't be able to maintain an aerobic pace for very long.

WALKING AND WEIGHT LOSS

Any kind of walk is good for you, so if you can't work up to an aerobic pace at first, it's fine to remain in the health or even the stroll category. Obviously, however, when you walk quickly you burn more calories than when you walk slowly. But although the intensity of your walk is important, it's more important that you keep moving for a long time than go at a fast pace. So 20 minutes at an aerobic pace isn't as good as an hour of a health walk; if you can't keep up a fast pace for very long, go slower for a longer amount of time. Your body doesn't start **burning fat** until about half an hour of activity, so if weight loss is your goal, you'll need at least 40 minutes to an hour of walking to make much of a difference.

If you want to **lose weight,** the best time to exercise is the morning. Your body burns sugar before it gets to using fat for energy. In the morning, you haven't built up as much sugar, so your body will start burning fat deposits faster. Morning work-outs will also jumpstart your metabolism for the whole day, causing you to burn more calories.

INCREASE YOUR STEPS THE EASY WAY

There are lots of ways you can incorporate walking into your daily routine. Try **parking further away** from your destination the next time you drive somewhere. Just an extra 100 yards can greatly increase your steps for the day. **Take walking breaks** at work instead of hanging out by the snack machine for an instant 10 minutes of exercise. Always **take the stairs** instead of the elevator. And organize your weekends around walking-based activities. Go to a craft fair or farmer's market where you'll have to walk to see everything. Or plan to meet up with friends for an evening stroll instead of talking over dessert.

If you try hard enough, you will find time to walk. Don't make any more excuses! We are a sitting nation, but you can break away from the norm. Get up and get moving!

HADJI'S TESTIMONY

I used to not exercise. I am 5'5" and weighed about 210 pounds. I had trouble breathing. I was on medication for my diabetes and high blood pressure. I also had high cholesterol, but I wasn't on any medicines for it. I went to see Dr. Kim for help with my fungal toenail problem. He said he could help me with the toenail if I wanted, but told me that it would clear up on its own if I got healthier. Dr. Kim then asked me if I wanted to get off my medications. He mentioned that his seminar could teach me how to change my lifestyle. Of course I want to get off my medicines, but I wasn't sure if the seminar would really work. Still, I decided to give it a try.

I went to the seminar and made the changes to my

diet and exercise habits that Dr. Kim suggested. I started exercising every day. At first, I could only do five minutes on my treadmill before I'd get winded. Within the first week, however, I was up to thirty minutes. Soon, I was doing one hour every day. I set up my treadmill in front of my TV, so I often didn't want to get off. Within three weeks into the program, I was off my diabetes and blood pressure medications with the approval of my general practitioner. I couldn't believe it!

Since the nine-week program, I'm off all my medications. My blood pressure has dropped as well. My resting heart rate used to be close to 100. Now, it's about 75. My cholesterol went down 78 points; my triglycerides went down 160 points, with my LDL level falling 40 points. I'm breathing better too. I've lost 25 pounds. I'm definitely a believer in Dr. Kim's program. I've been telling all my friends about it. It takes commitment, but I enjoy my new lifestyle and the results it has given me.

WHY NINE WELLNESS DOWEL EXERCISES?

I have done martial arts all my life. It started when I was a small and skinny kid who always got beat up in school. My mom didn't like that I was being picked on, so when I was eight, she enrolled me in Tae Kwon Do classes. She wanted me to learn to protect myself from the bullies. In junior high, I started learning Kendo, which is Japanese swordsmanship. In high school, I expanded to Kung Fu for a year. But it was not until I started to teach Tae Kwon Do in college that I really loved martial arts. I began learning Jujitsu, a Japanese grappling technique, at the same time.

When I was a martial arts instructor in college, one of my jobs was to teach the wrestling team. The guys on the team were all big and strong from lifting weights. As I taught them Tae Kwon Do, they taught me weight training and body building. I found that I really liked this aspect of exercise! By the time I went to medical school, I was working as a personal trainer and was heavily into body building. I lifted weights all the time.

After 25 years of weight training and 40 years of a variety of martial arts, I began wondering about what would be the ultimate exercise program. Eventually, I developed the nine dowel exercises, which work almost all the muscles in the body with a few simple stretches. The following exercises are the culmination of all my years of training in multiple athletic disciplines. They are both an aerobic and anaerobic workout, promoting principles of **stretching**, **strengthening**, proper **breathing**, and **balance**. They will increase your flexibility, improve your coordination, and promote strength and endurance. Here it is; the ultimate workout.

BASICS OF DOWEL EXERCISES

Before I describe each exercise, allow me to explain a few basic principles that will help you understand the routine better. The most important thing to remember when you're doing the dowel exercises is to maintain **correct posture.** Posture is the balance between your **abdominal muscles** and your **lower back muscles.**[268] Together, these muscle groups are called the **core muscles.** Concentrating on developing your core will enhance any fitness program.[269] A solid core will also help you maintain good posture and improve movement capability, two results which will help you in your daily life.[270] Every repetition of the dowel exercises will help build your core.

These routines may be the first time you breathe correctly in your whole life. Most people take shallow breaths all the time, but the dowel exercises require you to breathe fully. In fact, the average person takes 20,000 breaths each day, but the vast majority of these breaths are too shallow.[271] For the dowel exercise, inhale deeply, remembering that breathing in gives you life. Then, exhale fully, releasing any negative energy and frustrations. The following illustration shows the way you should be breathing. Your belly should expand when you take breaths in, not when you exhale.

With all of my exercises, I use a short, two-foot long dowel, as shown on page 133. Any stick will do as long as it's straight, has a medium thickness, and won't break when you apply pressure to it.

PREPARATION FOR DOWEL EXERCISES

Okay, now you're ready to get started! Here is how you should prepare for the exercises:

IT STARTS WITH GOOD BALANCE AND POSTURE. Keep your knees slightly bent and your feet spread shoulder width apart. Your body's weight should be on the balls of your feet. Don't strain your eyes while doing these exercises, in other words, keep your eyes soft. This will insure that you burn more stored fat rather than your stored sugar.[272]

PRACTICE BREATHING. Think of there being a triangle between your two hips and belly button. Now, imagine there's a ball inside that space. As you breathe in, you should feel the ball expanding. As you breathe out, it should feel like it's contracting.[273]. Think about the calming effects of breathing in and the cleansing effects of breathing out.[274] For each exercise, repetitions will be performed in 4-2-4 counts. Take four counts breathing in, hold your breath for two counts, and exhale over four counts. It is well known that the slower you exercise, the more strength you'll attain. So slow down and make each repetition count!

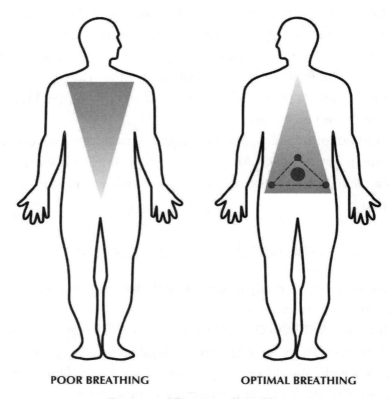

POOR BREATHING   **OPTIMAL BREATHING**

Proper and Improper Breathing

PERFORM ALL NINE OF THE EXERCISES, focusing on breathing and slow motion. When you inhale, squeeze your back muscles, or your "wings." When you exhale, squeeze your abdominal muscles. This method will develop your core.

START WITH TWO REPETITIONS THE FIRST WEEK. You can increase by one repetition each week thereafter. You should perform the dowel exercises before and after your walk, both as a warm up and cool down.

THE DOWEL EXERCISES

1. BOW

The first exercise will open up your chest and help stretch your spine. To do this stretch, start with your hands grasping the top of the dowel, about shoulder length apart. Then, inhale for four counts as you raise the stick over your head, arching your back slightly as shown in the picture. Squeeze your wings together and hold for two counts. You should feel the stretch at the back of your heels. To finish, exhale for four counts and bring the dowel back to the starting position in front of your body.

Exercise 1: BOW

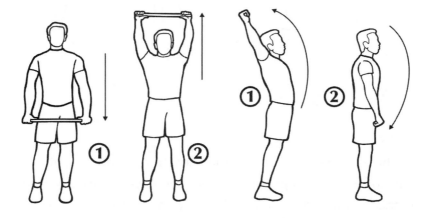

2. SIDE BEND

This exercise stretches the side of your body, but it will help your oblique abdominal muscles too if you remember to squeeze them when you bring your dowel up to the center. Begin this technique with both hands holding the dowel above your head. Bend to one side over four counts as you inhale. Hold for two counts and exhale as you return to the starting position, squeezing your abdominal muscles as you move. Repeat a second time, leaning to the other side.

Exercise 2: SIDE BEND

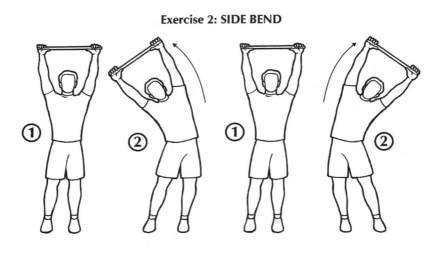

3. BACK

The back dowel exercise is the most important one for you to do often; it strengthens your upper back at first, but with practice it will work your middle and lower back too. Begin in the same position as the side bend, with your arms over your head holding your stick. Then, inhale for four counts as you bring the dowel behind your shoulders. Keep your wings tightly together as you hold for two counts. Finally, exhale and release the dowel to the starting position over four counts. You can do this exercise while you're **sitting down** in front of your computer at work. Every 20 minutes, do a few repetitions to fight the force of leaning forward and improve your back health.

In the back exercise, it's important to open up your chest

every time you bring the dowel behind your neck and shoulders. This way, you'll improve your posture by forcing the shoulders back. You'll get the most out of the exercise if your back is slightly arched when you're moving the stick down. Once you master the basic back exercise, try **rising up on your toes** with each downward motion. This is an advanced technique. Slightly rising on your toes will help you make the arch in your back more pronounced, which will make the muscles work harder to squeeze together.

Exercise 3: BACK

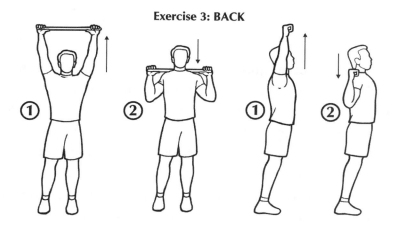

4. CHEST

This exercise strengthens the deltoid muscles around your shoulders, pectorals on your chest, and other middle back muscles. It's another good way to reverse the harm done by slouching. Begin this exercise with the dowel held directly in front of you at the level of your shoulders. Then inhale for four counts as you bring the stick into your chest, squeezing your back muscles together all the time. Hold this position for two counts, exhale, and release to the starting point over another four counts.

Exercise 4: CHEST

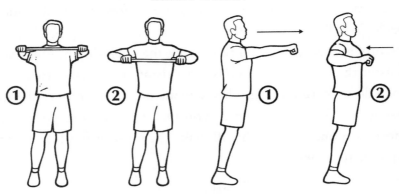

5. TWIST

The twist is another good exercise for your oblique abdominal muscles. Twisting helps improve the frontal rotation of your spine as well. For this exercise, start with the dowel in front of you and your arms at shoulder level. Turn to the left as you inhale for four counts; make sure your keep your arms at shoulder level, with your stomach in tight and your arms squeezed together. Hold the stretch on the left side for two counts and then return to the center position over a four-count exhale. Do the same movements while turning to the right side.

Exercise 5: TWIST

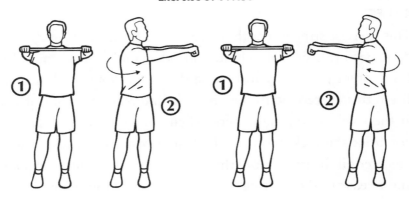

6. FRONT BEND

This exercise helps stretch out your hamstrings and lower back. To start, stand with your feet shoulder-width apart, holding the dowel loosely in front of you as shown. Over four counts, inhale as you bend forward, bringing the dowel as close to the ground as possible. Hold the stretch for two counts and then exhale as you return to the starting position.

Exercise 6: FRONT BEND

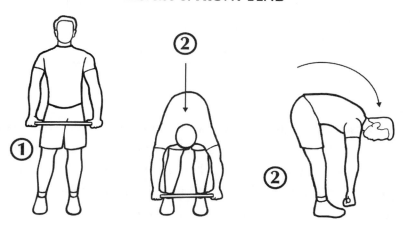

7. SQUAT

The squat works the lower back, thighs, buttocks, and leg muscles. Start this exercise standing with the dowel in front of you and your arms parallel to the floor. Over four counts, inhale as you squat to an almost seated position. You should keep your back straight, as shown in the picture. Hold the squat for two counts, and then exhale as you return to the start position over four counts.

Exercise 7: SQUAT

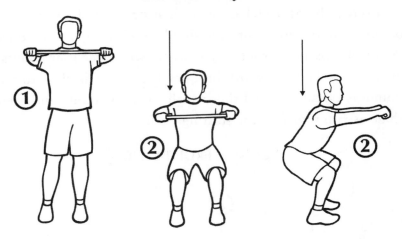

8. SCISSOR

The scissor stretch improves flexibility in your hip flexors, quadriceps and hamstrings. Start standing with your feet shoulder-width apart; the dowel should be resting low in both hands. Next, move the right foot back as you lunge deeply with the left leg and inhale for four counts. Keep your back straight to feel more of a stretch in your hip flexor. Press the dowel against

Exercise 8: SCISSOR

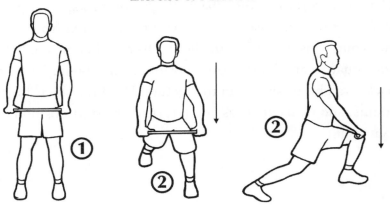

your front leg for support. Thrust your hips forward until you feel a stretch in your hip flexors. Remember to keep your front knee directly over your foot to prevent overly stressing your knee. Hold this stretch for two counts. Next, rise back to the starting position over four counts, exhaling as you come up. Repeat with the left leg moving back.

9. CALF

Use this exercise to help stretch your calf muscles and hamstrings. It's a lot like the scissor stretch above, except your back **heel doesn't come off the ground.** Start in the same position as the scissor stretch. Then, take four counts to inhale and move your right foot behind you into a lunge. Keep the heel of the right foot on the ground as you bend your left knee, making sure to keep the left knee over the left foot. Hold this stretch for two counts, and then return to the starting position over a four-count exhale. Repeat the whole movement, this time moving the left foot to the back and squatting with the right knee.

Exercise 9: CALF

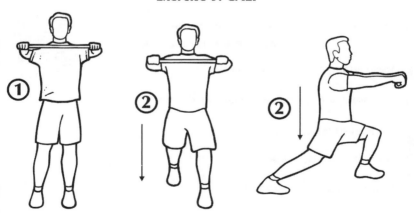

DOWEL EXERCISE BENEFITS

If you do these nine wellness dowel exercises every day, you'll see a huge improvement in your back strength before long. Start small—just two repetitions of each exercise will be enough at first. Just make sure you're doing each one correctly; keep your wings squeezed together, your arms straight, and your breathing patterns regular for the best results. Once you feel comfortable with the movements, gradually increase your repetitions to 10 of each exercise daily. Eventually, work up to doing them twice a day, and add in the back exercise whenever you have a few minutes—it's the most important for good back alignment.

Now that you know about my dowel exercises and walking program, put them both to work. You can't choose one or the other; both anaerobic strengthening and aerobic activity is required for a healthy life. It's best to do the dowel exercises before and after you walk. Do half your daily repetitions before you go out to walk as a warm up. Then, do the other half as a cool down set after you get back.

EXERCISE: PLANNING YOUR EXERCISES

When will I do anaerobic/strengthening exercise?

What kind of anaerobic/strengthening exercise will I do?

How long will I do this exercise?

When will I do aerobic exercise?

What kind of aerobic exercise will I do?

How long will I do aerobic exercise?

Remember, exercise is what keeps everything working together in your body. It's like the wind on earth—it keeps the cycle of elements in your body in motion. So don't hurt yourself by staying sedentary. Commit to exercising today, no matter how little you do to start. You'll get better in time, and you'll benefit no matter what.

SCHEDULE YOUR HEALTH

Look at the exercise schedule below. It shows that you should walk, do dowel exercises, and lift weights everyday. How do you compare? Draw your daily exercise activities in the blank chart on the right.

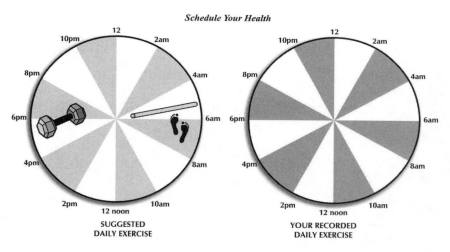

Schedule Your Health

SUGGESTED
DAILY EXERCISE

YOUR RECORDED
DAILY EXERCISE

EXERCISE WELLNESS SCORING CHART

Circle your exercise activities on the next chart. Mark how many steps you take daily and how many times you exercise weekly. If more of your circles are above the dotted line, give yourself one point.

Exercise Wellness Scoring Chart

Circle how many
steps you walk
each day

Circle how many
times per week
you exercise

LIFE

LIGHT

WELLNESS

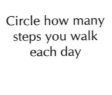

10,000 (80 minutes)

5 Times/Week

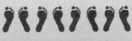
8,000 (60 minutes)

4 Times/Week

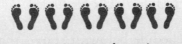

3 Times/Week

5,000 (40 minutes)

3,000 (25 minutes)

Twice/Week

DEATH

DARK

Once/Week

1,000 (8 minutes)

No Exercise

ILLNESS

Chapter 8
THE 7ᵀᴴ SECRET:
MOON

"REST, VACATE, RECREATE, RELATE, SET GOALS"

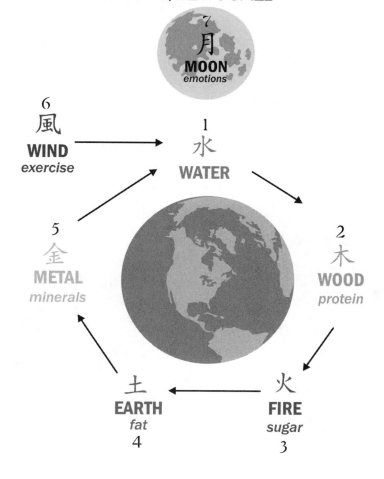

The moon is out and it is dark. It represents the emotions and thoughts in our heads, which are constantly taking us to darkness. The moon is the stress that makes us fat and dumb. It wreaks havoc on our system. Our emotional problems all started with authority figures in our childhood. And when we have emotional traumas and wounds, they govern us for the rest of our lives. We are rendered powerless when these inevitable negative emotions and thoughts control us. To overcome the darkness of the moon, we need to rest, vacate, recreate, relate, and set goals.

THE MOON IS OUT AND IT IS DARK

The moon pulls the earth with its gravity, creating tides. In our bodies, our heads represent the moon. Our **thoughts** and **emotions** can sway us just like the pull of the moon. Covered by a hard, thick skull, our heads do not allow a lot of light to get in. They represent the dark side of us all, places where our current **stress, past conditioning, and perceived limitations** are stored. As you can see in the illustrations, the influence

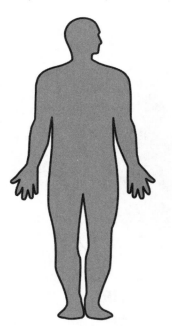

Darkness of Body

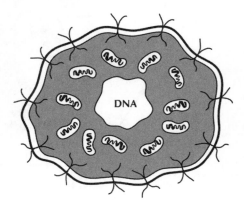

Darkness of Cell

of the moon makes our bodies and our cells filled with the darkness of poor health.

There's no denying that the things in our heads affect the way we live. They can control our behaviors and have a huge impact on our health. But we have to get them under control to live the best life. Remember: no natural light comes from the moon, no matter how much influence it has on the earth. Likewise, there's nothing fundamentally crucial about how our emotions affect us; our emotions are an invention of our own brains. But they do matter, all the same.

In this chapter, I'll talk about the three levels of consciousness and how each affects us. We'll spend the remainder of this book talking about these three levels and their corresponding elements of the universe: moon, sun, and heart. Later on in this chapter, I'll talk about stress, how it affects you, and what to do to overcome it. Finally, before ending this chapter about our heads, we will face our emotional wounds. After all this analysis, we'll be able to take control of the life-threatening and debilitating darkness that covers our lives.

THREE LEVELS OF CONSCIOUSNESS

Everything is connected, and everything is a part of something else. In this book, I've been talking about three "universes" time and time again. They are the solar system, the body, and the cell. Each of these things is self-contained, but each can also be broken down into smaller parts or could be considered a part of a larger whole. All three things—the cell, the body, and the solar system—mirror each other in their construction.

Each universe can also be divided into three parts, or levels of consciousness: the **subconscious**, the **conscious**, and the **superconscious**. Let's use our body to illustrate how these

Three Levels of Consciousness

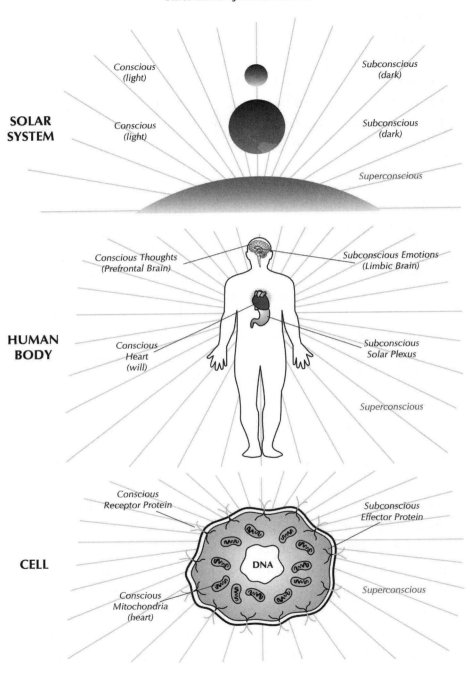

levels of consciousness play out. Follow along with the previous illustration.

First of all, the **subconscious** mind is like our autopilot mechanism. It represents the dark side of the earth and the moon. In our cells, the subconscious mind is equivalent to our effector proteins, which help carry out day-to-day activities and reactions. You can see the effector proteins in the illustration. The subconscious mind is equivalent to the solar plexus, a connection of nerves behind the heart. The limbic brain is also part of the subconscious mind. It's the program that runs our minds and bodies up to 99 percent of the time.[275] Like a recording machine, elements of the subconscious play back anything that has been impressed upon them.[276] The subconscious mind has about a million times the power of the conscious mind, which isn't always a good thing. For most people, the vast majority of the subconscious mind relates to negative feelings.[277]

In contrast to the subconscious mind is the **conscious** mind, which controls free choice and analytical thinking.[278] The conscious mind is like the bright side of the earth and moon. In our brains, the conscious thought is centered in the prefrontal cortex, the region responsible for concentration, planning, and decision making.[279] Our conscious mind can be compared to the receptor proteins in our cells, which make decisions about what substances can be allowed inside. Mitochondria are on the conscious level as well. They actively synthesize energy. Consciousness is also a part of your heart, the seat of free will.

Finally, the **superconscious** mind is the sun, which is the center of our being. This is the spiritual center that controls and governs our mind and body. As you can see, it radiates behind all levels of consciousness. Superconsciousness is really the mind of God, which is a perpetual power source because it radiates elements of God's character: omnipotence, boundless wisdom, beauty, and perfection. The superconscious mind is immeasurable and impossible for us to understand. However, we can examine the differences between the conscious mind and the subconscious mind. Look at the chart below to compare the two.[280]

DIFFERENCES In the CONSCIOUS and SUBCONSCIOUS MINDS	
CONSCIOUSNESS	**SUBCONSCIOUSNESS**
1 to 5 percent of our brain's usage	95 to 99 percent usage
Objective	Subjective
Waking	Sleeping
Surface of our brain (Prefrontal cortex)	Deep brain (Limbic system and brain stem)
Voluntary	Involuntary
Thoughts	Feelings/Emotions/Memory
Rational	Irrational
Personal/Decisions/Choice	Impersonal
Reasoning	Habitual
Desires/Wishes/Aspirations	Programs
Impressed	Expressed
Receives 40 bits of info per second	Receives 40 million bits of info per second

ARE YOU ALL STRESSED OUT?

Stress is one of the worst things for your health, but, unfortunately, many people are consumed by it. Some are so overrun by stress that they get sick. Experts estimate that 85 percent of illnesses are caused by stress.[281] About 100 million Americans suffer from some sort of stress-related illness, and 75 to 90 percent of all doctor's visits are stress related![282] These figures show that stress can take quite a toll of your life. Symptoms of **chronic stress** include irritability, loss of a sense of humor, worry, excessive eating and drinking, forgetfulness, aches and pains, nervousness, fatigue, and illness.[283]

WHAT CAUSES YOUR STRESS?

Many factors contribute to stress, and the primary causes vary from person to person. Some stress is more **physical** than emotional. Processed foods, dehydration, lack of exercise, lack of sleep, too much food, and eating too fast can all put stress on your body. **Emotional stress** can sometimes seem worse than physical stress, however. This kind of stress is caused by anger, fear, hunger, resentment, guilt, and inferiority. All of these feelings are controlled by your subconscious mind; you may not always know why you feel stressed out because it is an automatic response. A third kind of stress is **spiritual stress**. If you feel unconnected to your creator, you can experience huge levels of stress.

ANATOMY OF STRESS

Imagine walking down an alley in a big city at night. You feel a little nervous, but you keep going because the alley provides the shortest distance to your car. You hear someone walking behind you. Then, quickly, the person grabs you and puts a knife to your neck. How do you feel? More than likely, your heart would be racing, your hands would get clammy, and you would have trouble breathing. Those are the obvious, physical responses to your situation. Inside of you, more action would be taking place. About 30 negative hormones and 1400 chemical neurotransmitters would immediately be let loose into your blood stream.[284] At that moment, you would enter what is known as "fight or flight" mode.

The "fight or flight" reaction to stress all begins in your brain. When you perceive through your five senses that there is an impending threat to your life, your body turns on your **Reticular Activating System (RAS)**. There are 2 billion pieces of information being processed by your senses and transmitted to your RAS every second. When your RAS receives information, it filters it for value and relevance.[285] If alarming information is passed on to the RAS, it will send a signal to the hypothalamus, which will set a chain of stress-producing events in motion. First, the **hypothalamus** activates your **pituitary gland**. Then, the pituitary gland sends a signal to your **adrenal glands** to produce stress hormones. This system is called the HPA axis, which is an acronym for the three parts involved—hypothalamus, pituitary, adrenal.[286] When your stress hormones are released, blood is preferentially sent to your arms and legs instead of your main organs.[287]

STRESS WILL MAKE YOU FAT AND DUMB!

The stress hormones that your body produces might help you win a fight or run away quickly, but they're not good for you on a day-to-day basis. When you're stressed, your adrenal glands on top of your kidneys produce two main hormones: **adrenaline** and **cortisol**. They also churn out other neurotransmitters, known as **catecholamines**, which effectively "turn off" the concentration center of your brain. All three of these hormones can have negative effects on your health if they are in the blood stream long term.

ADRENALINE is released from the adrenal medulla, and when it gets in your blood stream, it will cause your blood pressure and heart rate to increase. It can also cause depression, anxiety, anger, a decreased sex drive, increased cholesterol, and diseases.[288] Adrenaline only stays in the blood for a short time, causing a sudden spike in energy followed by a draining crash.[289] This is why you feel good for a little bit when you're angry, scared, or stressed out. You're running on adrenaline, but when you crash, you feel terrible.

CORTISOL is another hormone released from the adrenal glands. More specifically, cortisol comes from the adrenal cortex. When it gets into your blood, cortisol prompts your body to release more fat and sugar that can be used as immediate energy.[290] This is good if you need to face your fear or run away quickly. But most of us don't need the reserves of energy that our bodies release in stressful situations, so the fat ends up being stored in deposits around the waists and hips.[291] The excess fat and sugar can also increase cholesterol levels. You'll probably feel unhappy and unmotivated with too much cortisol too; it is known to decrease the sex drive, testosterone, serotonin, and dopamine levels.[292]

Your adrenal glands also release other kinds of neurotransmitters known as **catecholamines**.[293] These messengers send signals to your brain to deactivate the prefrontal cortex, the area of the organ that controls concentration, planning, and analytical thinking. This is why you have trouble thinking clearly and making decisions when you're stressed out.[294] In other words, stress makes you dumb!

SLOW DOWN!

In these days of modern communication, stress seems almost inevitable. We don't have enough time to do everything that needs to be done.[295] In the past 20 years alone, time seems to have sped up dramatically due to new technology. Now, with cell phones and the Internet, we can get in touch with anyone anywhere almost immediately. Unfortunately, people's emotional reactions and stress levels have increased along with technology.[296]

We should all take a lesson from the time-old saying, stop and smell the roses! We need to stop multitasking. These days, everyone thinks it's okay to do more than one thing at one time, but that's not really true. Multitasking leads to fragmented attention and mental gridlock.[297] Most of us try to multitask because we think it will give us greater control over our lives. But we need to realize that we cannot control what happens to us. The only thing we can control is how we **perceive** what happens to us.[298]

Try to change the way you view stress. Instead of feeling overwhelmed and threatened by life's stressors, view them as an **opportunity for growth**.[299] This way, you won't experience the negative health effects of stress, but you'll still lead a fulfilled life.

IT ALL STARTED WITH YOUR CHILDHOOD

Think about what you perceive as stress. You might consider some things to be extremely stressful that other people don't think are a big deal. This is because your brain is programmed to give certain responses in certain situations. From the moment of your conception, your brain begins downloading different **programs** to run for the rest of your life. It's like getting a brand new computer and installing all the programs for the first time. Once you install the programs, your computer runs them automatically.

You keep downloading programs into your brain through the age of about seven. All of these programs are compiled to form your **subconscious mind**, which stays with you for the rest of your life. After you've reached the age of reason at about seven years old, you begin to develop your **conscious mind**. At this point, you can make decisions about whether to accept information as true or false.

Scientific studies have proven that your brain waves change as you grow through childhood. Infants less than a year old emit **delta waves**, the lowest frequency of brain activity. At about two years of age, children begin to emit more **theta waves**, which are the second-to-lowest category of brain emission.[300] These low-frequency brain waves correspond to more programmable states of being. In fact, hypnotists often drop their patients into states corresponding to delta or theta waves when they want to make an impression on them.[301] This is why young children absorb everything that their parents and other adults do. They develop their personalities and learn how to respond to stress in these impressionable, formative years. In fact, a five-year old child has more than 20,000 hours of parental tapes recorded in his or her brain![302]

It is not until they are between the ages of six and seven that children regularly give off **alpha waves,** which are equated to calm states of consciousness. This stage is when children first begin to have self awareness.[303] At around 12 years old, children start giving off **beta waves,** which are used in problem solving and focused thought.[304] It is not until these higher-frequency beta waves are produced that children are capable of everyday mental processing. In adults, beta waves are associated with everyday activity.[305]

BRAIN WAVES and CHILD DEVELOPMENT			
WAVE	Hz	AGE	STATE
γ Gamma	30+	>13	Excitement, Emotional State, Stress
β Beta	13-30	12-13	Everyday Activity, Stress, Conscious
α Alpha	8-12.9	6-7	Relaxation, Meditation, Subconscious
θ Theta	4-7.9	2	Deep Meditation: Sleep, Subconscious
δ Delta	2-3.9	0	Deep Sleep: Unconcscious

The programs that you record as a child are stored in your brain's **limbic system,** which is the emotional center responsible for fight or flight feelings. The limbic system also controls feeding and sexual emotions. Most of your **negative beliefs and programs** were incorporated into your brain at a young age, when you were most impressionable. These beliefs came from parents, other family members, friends, and teachers. Every day, these negative programs can be reinforced by all the people around you. You keep replaying the messages you first recorded, and if these messages are stress-producing or emotionally draining, you're making yourself sick!

NO WONDER YOU THINK YOU HAVE NO POWER

Every time your parents criticized you or scolded you as a child, you downloaded that information. It still affects you to this day. Your parents probably didn't know that their actions would make such a difference in your life, but everything they said and did helped shape the way you respond to emotional situations. Look over the following list of negative rules and messages you could have received as a child.[306] Did your parents ever say or imply these things?

These rules and messages are programmed into your **subconscious mind**. They make you feel powerless. Imagine having the message "you'll never accomplish anything" engrained in your mind. You would always have doubts about your abilities because, deep down, you'd be convinced that this message is

NO WONDER YOU THINK YOU HAVE NO POWER

NEGATIVE RULES	NEGATIVE MESSAGES
Don't express your feelings	You're not good enough
Don't get angry, upset, cry	Your needs are not all right with me
Do as I say, not as I do	Big boys don't cry
Avoid conflict	Act like a nice girl
Don't ask questions	You're stupid, bad, selfish
Don't discuss the family with outsiders	It's your fault
Be seen and not heard	You owe it to us
Don't talk back	I'm sacrificing myself for you
Don't contradict me	We won't love you if you...
Always be in control	You'll never accomplish anything
Always maintain the status quo	We wanted a boy/girl
Be dependent	I wish I never had you

the truth. When you are a slave to pre-programmed negative messages, you feel that you don't deserve the best things in life; your heath, your family, and your financial security can all suffer as a result.

THREE PARTS OF YOUR BRAIN

So far, we've touched on the outer layer of your brain, called the **conscious cortex**. This part of the brain is responsible for reasoning, planning for the future, and thinking. Unlike other parts of the brain, we have control over the prefrontal cortex. I also mentioned the **limbic system** of the brain, which is where the **subconscious messages** from your childhood are stored. This part of your brain is linked to your emotions and basic needs as well. You don't have control over what's stored in your limbic system, but you can change the way you respond to certain situations so the negative messages don't take over your life. You can see these parts of the brain in the illustration.

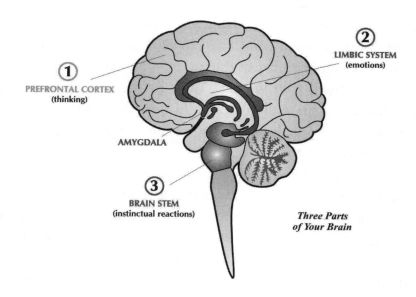

Three Parts of Your Brain

There's a third part of your brain that I haven't talked about yet. This is the **brain stem,** and it's responsible for the deepest part of your subconscious. Your brain stem controls your breathing, heart rate, stress response, and other automatic functions of your body.[307] As far as stress is concerned, one of the most important functions of the brain stem is maintaining equilibrium between your sympathetic and parasympathetic nervous systems. The sympathetic nervous system produces your stress response; your adrenal glands are part of this system. The parasympathetic nervous system, on the other hand, helps you rest and digest. When the sympathetic and parasympathetic nervous systems are imbalanced, you can develop diseases.[308] Your brain stem works hard to keep these systems in balance, but it isn't always successful.

EMOTIONAL TRAUMA/WOUNDS

Emotional trauma is what happens when you absorb negative rules and messages. Usually, emotional trauma can be traced to one event that had a profound impact on you. Maybe your parents scolded you for something you didn't do, or possibly you were embarrassed in front of a crowd. Emotional trauma can result from any number of things, and you may not even realize what caused your wounds. Most people have experienced emotional trauma multiple times in their lives, and for many people, these wounds become so deeply entrenched that they affect everything they do.

Many of our **emotional wounds** are stored in the limbic system, the part of our brains that controls the basic functions that I mentioned above. Unfortunately, the limbic system also serves as a sort of storage center for trauma. There's a part of your brain known as the **amygdala,** and it's where your emotional memories get stored. Interestingly, the amydgala is located right in the middle of the limbic area, so emotional memories and the limbic system's instinctual responses are closely related.

When you experience something traumatic, your amygdala receives input with a very high emotional value. It goes into panic mode because it is overwhelmed by the overly emotional data. The amygdala cannot send this information to the rest of your brain, so it stores it for long-term memory.[309] From these emotions, we learn how to react to similar situations we encounter in the future. So if we experience something traumatic that makes our limbic systems signal "fight," then we'll learn to always give that response in similar situations.

People whose limbic systems signaled "fight" at a young age tend to deal with trauma with anger. "Flight," on the other hand, translates to rejection, fear and guilt. Throughout lives, little things can trigger the emotional responses that were first buried in the amygdala. Our brains don't know how to process trauma, so as a defense mechanism, we always go back to what we know—either anger or rejection. I will tell you more about these two traumatic responses in detail further on. Although we know that trauma is associated with emotional responses, there's no formula for predicting your behavior or your emotions when you experience something that reminds you of your past pain. You have to look inside yourself to find the answers to all of your current problems.[310]

When you suffer from deep emotional trauma, you cannot have healthy relationships because you become **selfish**. Everything is all about you. You are constantly caught up in preserving your image of control and trying to avoid facing your wounds. Deep-rooted trauma also causes you to lose vitality—your desires, self assuredness, peace, and spiritual power. At least 40 percent of people have experienced some kind of serious abuse early in life, be it physical or sexual.[311] This kind of trauma drastically affects their daily lives. It's devastating.

LOVE SICK

You are designed to receive love to be healthy. When you don't receive an adequate amount of love, you get sick. I call this "love sick." The kind of love I'm talking about comes from the many relationships in your life: your relationship with God who designed you, created you, and loves you no matter what; your relationship with your spouse and loved ones; your relationship with your coworkers, who you spend most of your day with; and your relationship with your authority figures, usually your parents, who influenced you growing up. You need to receive enough love from these relationships to sustain you and help you thrive in life.

Have you ever been hurt by someone you loved? If so, you know what it feels like to be love sick. It is so painful and sickening to go through. Love is the glue of the relationships you have in your life; it's what keeps these—often voluntary—connections sticking together. If you fail to be connected by this glue, you will experience separation. However, when you use the glue to keep your relationships together, you won't be sick anymore.

Being love sick is the cause of many illnesses that we suffer. But the cure is easy: once you have plenty of love in your life, it will heal all of your emotional wounds. Love plays a huge role in your quality of life. It gives life by its nature, neutralizing everything bad you experience. It fills up every dead space with physical, emotional, mental, and spiritual goodness. Love is what transforms rejection to **dedication**, anger to **compassion**, hunger to **intimacy**, fear to **trust**, inferiority to **humility**, and guilt to **forgiveness**.

EMOTIONAL TRAUMA FROM
YOUR AUTHORITY FIGURES

By far the biggest source of emotional trauma is the kind inflicted by **authority figures,** most often parents. Other people with influence in children's lives can also cause damage, however; sometimes, teachers, coaches, grandparents and older siblings are the ones that spark emotional trauma. The truth is, almost every child suffers emotional trauma brought on by authority figures, and these people may not even know they're doing harm. All it takes is a negative comment, a comparison to another child, an offhand complaint, and a child will be marked for life. The emotional reflexes will generate a response, and the child will start building walls, either internally or externally. I'll talk more about building walls further in this chapter.

The problem with authority figures all boils down to one simple equation: love equals happiness. Imperfect love equals trauma. And "imperfect love" doesn't mean that the authority figure doesn't care about a child. In many cases, that's not true at all. Instead, **no love** refers to what the child perceives—absences, divorce, unplanned pregnancies. There's also **painful love,** the kind that's abusive or shameful. Finally, **wrong love** is when an authority figure expresses his or her love in a harmful way, like punishing children as a dictator or overprotecting them. All three of these flawed kinds of love can form deep impressions.

NO LOVE

Let's start with the **no love** scenario. I experienced this kind of trauma as a young boy. My father, a major authority figure in a child's life, left when I was four years old. I didn't know why he went away at the time. Part of me thought that it was to get away from me and the family. Later, I learned that he left to find work. Still, I was traumatized. His absence affected me greatly; I felt like it was my fault, in a sense. Understandably, I reacted with a defense mechanism—in my case, it's a combination of anger and rejection. It's like my brain told me to fight and run away at the same time.

Any kind of **absence** affects a child and can be considered emotional trauma.[312] Even when parents don't mean to harm their children with their absence, it's usually wounding for the kids. When authority figures are gone, there's no one around to give love. Anger, rejection, or hunger defenses can result.

Divorce is another version of the no love trauma from an authority figure. I will tell you right now, divorce always affects children, no matter how well it's handled. It guarantees that at least one parent will be absent all the time. There are worse things than divorce, no question, and it could be worse for a child to be around two parents who are constantly fighting. But a divorce, from a child's point of view, means that parents are there but not there. They might live across town but never be seen except on weekends. Children feel like their non-custodial parents are too busy to see them. Even though most parents hate to think that their divorce causes their children problems, unfortunately, it does. A divorce is traumatizing to kids.[313]

The no love version of trauma also includes **unwanted pregnancy**. Children may not remember their time in the womb, but they can still be scarred from things that happened to them then. I had a good friend who always felt unloved by his mother. He couldn't figure out why, since his childhood had been relatively good. It turned out that his parents didn't want to have a baby when he was conceived. His mother had tried to kill him in the womb. Believe me; that made a difference. My friend absorbed this trauma and it affected him all his life. If you feel like there's love missing in your life, ask your parents if they had planned for you to be born. You may find that unwanted pregnancy is the root of all your emotional issues.[314]

PAINFUL LOVE

The second kind of trauma brought on by authority figures is **painful love**. This happens most often when parents or other people in power abuse children emotionally or physically. They don't know how to interact with their kids, so they hurt them. Most often, **verbal abuse** brings fear; **physical abuse** brings anger. My mother was verbally harsh on my sisters and me when we were children. Looking back now, I see that she was stressed out about raising a family without her husband around. But at the time, it was horrible. She would yell at us, and she would always tell my sisters that they weren't good enough. Of course that kind of talk makes an impression on kids. How could it not?

Painful love also occurs when parents **favor children**. Sometimes, one child will seem to be perfect, while the others have trouble in school or in social situations. It's easy for parents to favor their children in these situations. They think they're motivating them by rewarding the achieving sibling, but really, they are wounding all parties involved. Preferential treatment will, undoubtedly, result in emotional problems.[315]

Another form of painful love is **shameful** authority figures. This most often occurs when parents are seen as inadequate in children's eyes. They may be too old, too uneducated, or too poor compared to other parents. The children become ashamed. It's especially bad when parents try to overcompensate for their faults, which can lead to the children feeling frustrated in addition to being embarrassed.

WRONG LOVE

In addition to no love and painful love, many times authority figures give children **wrong love**. They think they're helping their kids' development, but really, they're hindering it. Wrong love happens when the way an authority figure loves his or her children is flawed. Even the best authority figures love their children the wrong way sometimes. But if you have children or interact with them on a regular basis, you can make a conscious effort to give good love as often as possible. Don't compare children, don't play favorites, and don't make conditions for your love.

Two common forms of wrong love among parents are **spoiling** and **dictating**. Honestly, both kinds are bad, but if you have to be one or the other, it's better to be a dictator than a spoiler. Spoiled kids get mixed messages. They expect to get everything they want, and when they don't get their way in the real world, they're paralyzed. The common response to this emotional trauma is anger; people are frustrated when they can't get what they want. Parents who act like dictators elicit the opposite reaction from their children; instead of getting angry, kids with overbearing parents tend to cower in fear. They build their walls internally because they've learned to be afraid of authority.

FRANK'S TESTIMONY

I was in prison for 27 years of my life. I have a few children that I didn't get to build a relationship with because of my incarceration. One day, while I was in prison, I tried to escape. I ended up falling from a water pipe that was seven stories high. I crushed my heel and have had trouble walking ever since. After I got out of prison, I saw many doctors to try to fix my heel problem. Eventually, I found Dr. Kim. He treated my heel and told me about his seminar series. I decided to go.

At the seminar, we talked about emotional trauma. Dr. Kim told us that most of our problems start in childhood. He asked us to think of any traumatic experiences we had as kids. Thinking about my past in the seminar made me realize that all of my problems could be traced to one moment when I was a boy. I discovered that my criminal life began when my father punished me one afternoon. I stood up to a bully at school and refused to give him any money when he asked. I beat him up. Later, the bully's mother showed up at my parents' door. She told my dad that I had beat up her son. My dad didn't ask me about the situation at all; he just started hitting me as a punishment. He made me kneel on rice for an hour. I got angry. I was so upset that my dad would punish me without asking for my side of the story. I felt rejected and became rebellious. So I left home and started doing bad stuff. I rebelled against all authorities that told me what to do. That's how I ended up in and out of jail.

Until I met Dr. Kim, I never knew why I did the things I did. In the seminar, I realized that because of the emotional trauma that we suffer from authority figures, our lives can change. I loved my dad, but his actions had a huge impact on me. Now, I know that I need to develop relationships with own children. Since the seminar, I have had a much better relationship with my kids, and I plan to keep it up.

DEFENSE MECHANISMS

When I talk about **walls,** I am taking about the way we form our personalities. Your walls are your **defense mechanisms;** they're the way you respond in difficult situations. From the moment you were conceived, you started building your "self." Along the way, you built walls too. Think of the walls as the way you define yourself; they shape your personality and your responses to tough situations. But whenever you experience trauma, your walls get built a little off kilter. Instead of being straight, they're angled either toward you or away from you as a defense mechanism.

If you're one whose instinctual response to trauma is **anger,** then your walls points away from you. You blame other people for your problems, as demonstrated by your quick temper. But if you use **rejection** as your response, then your walls are built inward. You tend to blame yourself for everything that goes wrong. Depending on your personality, at any one time you could be either on the rejection side or on the rebellion/anger side. The way you respond to difficult situations is like a pendulum that is constantly swinging from one side to the other.

Regardless of how you respond to it, trauma tends to create the same patterns in lives. Where there is trauma, there is **no inner peace, no healthy relationships** and **no vitality.** Inner peace comes when we accept who we are; but with trauma, we can't accept ourselves. We either deny anything that we do wrong and build our walls outward, or we internalize everything and build inward-facing walls. Either way, we're not comfortable. We can't have healthy relationships where trauma is involved either. Trauma makes us **selfish;** we're only concerned about how we will be affected in life. Finally, trauma undermines vitality. With trauma, we become like animals without passion and without motivation—the opposite of vitality.

REJECTION AND REBELLION/ANGER

Our walls define our personality, and they are either tilted inward or outward. Typically, **introverted** people build their walls inward with rejection; they blame themselves when something goes wrong. In contrast, **extroverted** people build their walls toward the outside in anger, blaming the rest of the world for their problems. Think about yourself: which way do your walls face? Do you tend to respond to sticky situations with anger or with rejection? These are difficult questions to answer, and it takes some serious introspection to find out what kind of person you are.

People whose emotional problems stem from rejection blame themselves for problems; they keep their emotions hidden internally. This is the start of all emotional trauma and wounds.[316] Often, rejection manifests itself as **depression**, and in extreme cases it can lead to suicide. Common feelings associated with rejection include sadness, self-pity, self-hatred, apathy, inferiority, insecurity, failure, and guilt.

My father is a prime example of someone who responds to trauma with **rejection**. He was born in Japan in 1934, during the Japanese occupation of Korea. My grandfather was a ceramic maker who was sent to Japan to make ceramics during this time. My father's mother died from lung disease when he was just five years old, and my grandfather remarried and had six more children. My father and his brother were abused by their new stepmother, especially after my grandfather went back to Korea to work. She favored her own children over them. My father was severely beaten for eating too much all the time. This lack of love and abuse left my father feeling rejected. He still cries every time he talks about that time. As brilliant as my father is, he hardly talks. My mother always tells him to express himself, but he is more comfortable not talking. He always had business partners who took advantage of him. In fact, one time his partner kicked him out of a company he had set up! People on the rejection side like my father have no power to fight back in conflict. They simply hide.

Anger, on the other hand, is associated with rebellion. Rebellion is actually an expressed form of anger.[317] And anger is a negative energy generator.[318] People who respond to trauma with anger display their emotions externally. They blame others for their problems. In extreme cases, anger reactions can lead to homicide. Symptoms associated with anger defenses include resentment, conceit, elation, superiority complexes, competitiveness, overbearing attitudes, and overpowering personalities.

People who use anger as a defense mechanism begin to depend on it. A prime example of this is my mother. She was born in 1939 in the southwest part of Korea. When she was growing up, very few people could afford food, yet alone an education. Her father was an alcoholic who beat his wife daily. My mother was in constant fear. She was the youngest of eight children. Her father did not beat her, but her oldest brother beat her often for not working on the farm all the time. Tired of being abused, she left home at 17 and went to work in Seoul, the capitol of Korea. Some of her brothers later became wealthy, but they refused to help her. She became so resentful and angry at her siblings that she stopped communicating with her whole family. To make matters worse, the Korean War broke out in 1950 when she was 11 years old. I grew up listening to her rant about her anger toward all of her family.

Although we don't like to admit our flaws, all of us tend to fall into either the rejection or anger groups. Think about which symptoms match up with your personality. Do you have more rejection or more anger?

EXERCISE: REJECTION OR REBELLION

Which side do you have more of - rejection or rebellion?

Why do you think you fall more into this category?

Can you recall a specific incident that affected you in that way? What happened?

Why did your authority figure act that way? If you don't know, commit to finding out.

Now that you know whether you have been conditioned to respond with anger or rejection to tough times, you can try to control these responses. In general, it's not what happens to you that elicits a response, but how you **perceive** it. For example, if you get angry when your husband or wife forgets something, it might not be because the thing was very important. More likely, you perceive the situation differently from what really happens. Maybe you think your spouse doesn't care about you because he or she forgot your needs. Or possibly it seems to you that your husband or wife is purposely trying to hurt your feelings. Maybe neither of these things are true, but if you perceive that they are, you will respond accordingly. Once you're healed of your emotional wounds, you stop caring so much about what happens. Your perception is no longer skewed by your ingrained trauma.

HUNGER AND FEAR

Hunger and fear are two more emotional responses to a lack of love in childhood, but they're less about trauma and more about overall closeness. Both have to do with intimacy issues, but in different ways.

Hunger is a survival mechanism. Our brains tell us we're hungry so we eat. We need to satisfy our hunger to be happy; otherwise, it's constantly in the forefront of our minds. Emotional hunger is just like physical hunger, except that it's not food that is desired, but **intimacy**. Emotional intimacy happens when we share our deepest thoughts and feelings with others. When you are emotionally hungry, only love and intimacy can fill your void. People who hunger for intimacy can't get past their internal walls, so they overcompensate. They depend too much on other people because there's no true intimacy in their lives. You know people like this—the kind who always try to please everyone, who go out of their way to be friendly. But people can't reciprocate when we overdo friendliness, so hungry types are perennially disappointed. They are hurt easily by others.[319] Understandably, people who hunger for intimacy often try to satisfy their hunger with an **addiction**. Food is a big problem for hungry people; the hunger for intimacy can feel like physical hunger, but it's never satisfied because what's really needed is true closeness.

My wife is a good example of someone with emotional hunger. Her father was a minister who was very busy with church work all his life. Her parents had to constantly visit church members and were not around to take care of her much. When she was 11 years old, her father left for the United States to set up a church. My wife finally came to the United States when she was 22, but she had been separated from her father during the years she needed him most. Her mother favored her older brother and let out her frustrations on my wife. Due to this lack of love and intimacy from her parents, my wife became overly attached to her friends. She is always overly nice to people, and people take her for granted. They don't appreciate her. She expects a lot from people because she gives a lot to them. Unfortunately, most people don't appreciate people or things when they are freely given! She also has rejection issues, so she has a tough time confronting people. This makes her relationships much worse. And it all started with hunger.

Fear, on the other hand, is a result of instability in intimacy. Fearful types may have had intimacy at one time and then lost it. People with fear worry too much about what other people think, so instead of searching for intimacy, they do all they can to avoid it. Anticipation gets the most of them, and they get stressed. Fearful people may blame others for their intimacy problems; they think the world is out to get them and hide from it to avoid getting hurt. Interestingly, people with fear have problems with addiction just like people with hunger, and for similar reasons. People with fear secretly crave intimacy, and they try to fulfill their desire with addictions to things like alcohol, TV, money, and drugs. They want these things to provide them with security, which they can't have in their real lives because they don't allow themselves to take risks.

MY FEAR

Fear is something that I have to deal with a lot. My father went to Vietnam to work when I was four years old. It was difficult for him there, so he could not support us much financially. My mother had to raise three children by herself. She was a strong woman, and she disciplined us relentlessly. She said she did not want us to be called "fatherless" children. I remember when I was around six or seven years old, she was counting money in front of me. She laid out all the cash in front of her and counted, dividing some for food, some for school, and some for clothes. When she was done, she would count again. Then again and again for hours as if more money would miraculously appear. She sighed in between each count, and I knew that we didn't have enough. At that point, I decided I would work really hard to get more money so she wouldn't have to count so many times.

This fear of poverty has been driving me all my life. When I came to the United States when I was 16, I was already a sophomore in high school. High school was not easy, but I managed somehow. The problems came when I went to college. I did not understand at least half of what the professors were saying. I followed every professor after class and spent another hour finding out what they had said. One time, I wanted to do so well on a test that I stayed up for seven days in a row! At the end of my sleepless stint, I was hospitalized with an IV in my arm for a week. Amazingly, some of my professors came to visit me in the hospital. They were wondering what had happened to the Korean boy!

I had two part-time jobs when I was in college and a full-time job as a weight trainer when I was in medical school. I was driven by my fear of failure and poverty. I could not stop to think. I just kept working harder. When I got married, my wife began to notice how I worked day and night. She said, "Honey, why are you working so hard? You have enough to spend. Why don't you get some rest?" But I couldn't rest. I have been chased by this huge lion of fear, which I felt was about to eat me alive. I was addicted to work. That is the danger of fear.

Both hunger and fear can be cured with real **intimacy**. We have to remember that in order to be intimate with someone we have to make the first move. If you have problems with hunger or fear, try to look at your situation objectively. Make an effort to be truly intimate with a friend or partner; this will mean exposing the deepest part of yourself. The person you want to share with may have his or her own issues, so don't get discouraged if you feel like intimacy is hard to achieve. It will take time, but eventually, you'll both get through your walls and become truly close.

Before you can try to eliminate fear or hunger you have to identify whether these emotional problems affect you. Think about the following questions:

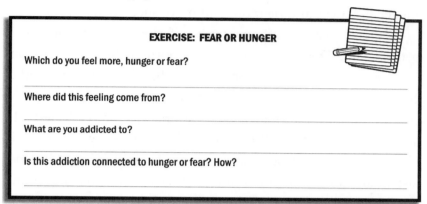

EXERCISE: FEAR OR HUNGER

Which do you feel more, hunger or fear?

Where did this feeling come from?

What are you addicted to?

Is this addiction connected to hunger or fear? How?

As with anger and rejection, hunger and fear can often be traced to a specific event that took place during childhood. It can take lots of work to identify the root of your hunger or fear, and even more effort to recondition your programmed response, but it's worth it to make it a priority to end your fear or hunger. Only then will you be able to have a stable, satisfying life.

INFERIORITY AND GUILT

Inferiority and **guilt** are both results of the four traumas listed above—rejection, anger, hunger, and fear. A person with an inferiority complex has no value of self. And, unfortunately, at least one third of people have this condition.[320] Personally, I think that it affects more people; we just don't know about it.

Feelings of inferiority often lead to an **obsession with perfection**. I'm a good example of this. I am a perfectionist who thrives on doing things right. I have a tremendous inferiority complex when it comes to doing things right and being better than anyone else. I believe this came from my fear and hunger. My need for perfection makes my life very tiring. I have so much to read and learn, so many seminars I want to attend, and so many places I want to go visit. I want to have bigger and bigger practices and be more and more successful.

My two sisters suffered from inferiority when they were growing up. They always felt less important than me. This was not because I was superior to them but because my mother brainwashed them. In Korean culture, males are preferred, so my mother favored me over my sisters. No matter how bad I was, my mother told all my friends how I was a great son. My sisters, on the other hand, never received compliments. My older sister, Sue, was brilliant in school but never was given any credit. And my younger sister, Jackie, was adventurous, outgoing, and had lots of friends, but she was only told she was not lady like. Anything I did right was praised and recognized, but none of their good qualities ever were.

Guilt is usually a result of failure. People tend to dwell on past failures for too long and too hard. They can't forgive themselves or others for shortcomings, and they are overly critical. I feel totally guilty when I don't get things done or when I fail at certain things. I become overly sensitive about my failures. This is debilitating because I don't want to try many new things in life due to possible failures. I don't believe that I am good enough many times. That is why this book has taken me seven years to complete. Most of my seminar attendees have told me that I need to write a book. I've been hearing that for years. But I didn't think I knew enough to write a book.

Consider your own life. Do you ever feel inferior or guilty? Honestly answer the next questions to find out. Then, you can start working to overcome these feelings.

EXERCISE: INFERIORITY OR GUILT

Do you feel inferior often and when?

Do you always compare yourself to others?

Write down your shameful experiences or failures:

COPING WITH EMOTIONAL TRAUMA

How do you deal with your fear, hunger, rejection, anger, inferiority, and guilt? Recognizing that you have these problems and identifying their causes is a first step. But to cope with emotional wounds on an everyday basis, you need to make your life more fulfilling. There are five things you can do to increase your satisfaction: rest, vacate, recreate, relate, and set goals.

REST

When the moon comes out, it's time to wind down. Your body and mind need rest to recuperate after a day's worth of focus and work. Contrary to popular belief, each day starts when you go to bed and get **sleep**, not when you wake up in the morning. The same can be said for each week out of the year; a week starts on Sunday, the day of rest when you relax before your journey through the next six days. Each year starts in winter, a time for dormancy and rest when the earth gets ready for the liveliness of the rest of the year. You were in your mother's womb to prepare for your journey through life. All of these examples have one thing in common—rest.

It is of the utmost importance that you rest properly. And

173

although sleep is the most important type of rest, other forms are necessary as well. You need to have time to wind down and relax each day for good health.

YOU ARE A TIME MACHINE

There is a **rhythm of life**, a rhythm which encompasses all things. And you are dancing with it. The earth, the moon, and the sun are dancing with this rhythm too. Each is perfectly coordinated: the earth rotates on its axis every 24 hours, creating one day; the moon rotates around the earth every 29.5 days; the earth rotates around the sun every 365.2 days, or once each year.[321]

In your own body, you are guided by a master clock of sorts. This "clock," called the **suprachiasmatic nucleus** (SCN), is located within the hypothalamus, a small gland in your brain.[322] The SCN signals your body when to release melatonin, a hormone associated with sleep, and other neurotransmitters into your blood stream.[323] These hormones tell your body when it's time to wake up and when to go to bed, keeping you on a regular cycle. Sunlight is what makes your internal clock work; it entrains the SCN, which coordinates hormone release with the light of day.[324]

JET LAG AND SHIFT LAG

Many people travel to different time zones all the time. Excessive travel is required for some jobs, but it's not a good thing for your body. It breaks the rhythm of life. People who travel to another time zone need to take time for recuperation after their journeys. It takes one day to get used to just one time zone change.[325] You can't always avoid traveling, but you can make an effort to be gentle on your body when you do it. Give your-self the rest you deserve!

As bad as jet lag can be for your health, **shift lag** is worse. It's like having constant jet lag. Shift lag occurs when people don't sleep during normal resting hours, usually because of work. This throws your body way out of whack. More than 20 percent of the global work force performs night shifts, and, in America, more than 15.2 million workers work night hours.[326] This is devastating to these workers' health because it means a constant disruption of circadian rhythms. Breaking the rhythm of life by working night shifts can cause multiple health conditions, espe-cially heart, stomach, and mental problems.[327] If you must work night shifts, you need to stay on a regular sleep schedule every day of the week, even on the weekends. This will ensure that your body doesn't experience the havoc of shift lag.

SLEEP YOUR WAY TO HEALTH

Sleep is by far the best way to rest. It's important for your health because it allows your subconscious mind to work without the interference of your conscious mind.[328] When you sleep, your brainwaves slow down to theta or delta levels, allowing your brain to take a break from the more taxing, higher-frequency processes. Sleep promotes learning, improves proficiency at tasks, and sustains emotional well being. It also improves mem-ory, creativity, concentration, and alertness.[329] The bottom line: you need sleep to function.

SLEEP EQUALS EXERCISE

I have found that sleep offers the same benefits as exercise. This doesn't mean that you can forgo exercise for more sleep, however. What it does mean is that when done regularly and in balance, both sleep and exercise can drastically improve your health. Both increase the production of **growth hormone,** which helps fuel vitality. Both also boost your immune system, increase your brain function, and up your sex drive. And sleep and exercise can help fight health problems too; they have been shown to decrease cortisol production, reduce signs of aging, and fight against incidents of disease.[330]

LACK OF SLEEP

Before Thomas Edison invented the light bulb in 1879, people slept an average of 10 hours each night.[331] Now, most of us get less than seven hours. In fact, the current national average for nightly sleep is 6.9 hours.[332] This is not enough! You need a minimum of seven to nine hours of sleep each night, and some people need even more to function fully.[333]

Insomnia is becoming a serious epidemic![334] Lack of sleep is rampant, with 50 to 70 percent of Americans suffering from insufficient nightly rest. Sleep problems do more than just leave people feeling groggy. Insomnia is costly. More than 42 million sleeping pills are prescribed each year, which takes a toll on personal finances. Also, over $100 billion is lost each year because of lack of sleep. This money is eaten up by lost productivity, medical expenses, sick leave, and property and environmental damages.[335] As you can see, insufficient sleep definitely takes its toll.

WHAT CAUSES INSOMNIA?

Multiple factors contribute to sleep problems. Some can be controlled with lifestyle changes, but others occur naturally with some people. A few of the biggest causes of insomnia are **stress, anxiety, pain, caffeine, medicines, alcohol, processed foods, low-carb diets, exercising too late at night, going to the bathroom in the middle of the night,** and **bad pillows or mattresses.**[336] When you follow my advice about diet and exercise in this book, you will probably find that your insomnia will go away naturally.

STAGES OF SLEEP

When you sleep, your subconscious mind takes over. But not all types of sleep are the same. There are two main types of sleep that fill our nights: **REM sleep,** which is when we dream, and **non-REM sleep,** which is also known as quiet sleep. During REM sleep, your mind is restored to its full potential. REM sleep also improves your ability to learn and store memories.[337] About every 90 minutes a sleeper enters REM sleep, meaning that most of us have three to five dreams a night.

REM sleep helps restore your mind, but non-REM sleep is what is good for your body. In non-REM sleep, your brainwaves are at low frequencies; alpha, theta, and delta waves are common. During these sleep stages your body releases growth hormones. Tissue grows and damage is repaired in your body. Work is done to improve your immune system too.[338] Both REM and non-REM sleep are important. Together, they heal your body and mind.

TYPES OF SLEEPERS

You've probably noticed that your sleep habits are different from those of other people. That is completely normal. There are many different kinds of sleepers in the world because people have different circadian rhythms. Some people go to sleep early and get up before dawn; they are called **larks**. Other people don't feel like going to bed until well after midnight and sleep until late in the morning; these types are called **owls**. Most people, however, have internal clocks that tell them to go to bed between 10:30 and 11:30 p.m. and wake up between 6:30 and 7:30 a.m.[339] Your own personal sleep schedule is called your **chronotype**.

The number of hours that people need to sleep varies too. You might think that you can function with just a few hours of sleep each night, but the truth is you probably can't. Only about five percent of people can comfortably get less than five hours of sleep each night. These people won't feel groggy or be less productive if they don't sleep much. On the contrary, about five percent of people need more than 10 hours of sleep each night to feel their best! For most people, however, seven to nine hours is ideal.[340]

HOW TO GET BETTER SLEEP

If you have trouble sleeping or feel that your sleep isn't satisfying, try the following suggestions for improving your sleep time.

EXERCISE. When you exercise, your body produces serotonin, which will help you sleep better.[341] You'll also use up some of your energy and feel more tired.

KEEP A REGULAR SLEEP SCHEDULE so your body gets used to sleeping and waking at similar times. Try not to deviate from your schedule too much over the weekend.

DECREASE THE NOISE in your bedroom. This might mean sealing your doors and windows or wearing earplugs.

BLOCK ANY BEDROOM LIGHT. When it's dark, your body produces melatonin, which helps you go to sleep.

DECREASE YOUR CAFFEINE CONSUMPTION, especially late in the day.

DECREASE YOUR ALCOHOL CONSUMPTION. Alcohol is a stimulant, not a sedative.

PRACTICE RELAXATION TECHNIQUES like deep breathing, visualization, meditation, prayer, biofeedback, acupuncture, and hot baths.[342] Try these techniques about an hour before bed to prepare your body for sleep.

DON'T SLEEP HUNGRY. Try eating a bedtime snack to help keep your blood sugar constant throughout the night. A light snack of fruit or nuts works well.[343]

KEEP YOUR BEDROOM CLEAN. Looking at clutter won't help you relax.

Make sure your **mattress and pillows** are comfortable.

PRACTICE BEING IN THE PRESENT MOMENT. Don't feel guilty about the past or worry about the future.[344]

POWER NAPS ANYONE?

In many countries around the world, people take a **siesta** every afternoon. All of the stores and businesses shut down for a few hours so people can take naps . . . what a concept! We could all learn from the siesta model. It makes sense to take a short nap in the afternoon because we are designed to sleep twice each day. Taking naps is proven to increase alertness and enhance performance throughout the day.

You will know when you need a nap. Most people start to feel sleepy in the afternoon, which signals that a short power nap is in order. Based on the rhythm of life, our bodies usually need naps between 2 and 3 p.m. For most people, a 10- to 30-minute nap is all that's needed to feel rejuvenated.[345]

NATURAL SLEEP AIDS

Don't resort to chemical sleeping pills if you have problems with insomnia. These sleep aids are overly processed and aren't good for your health. They can be addictive, and some are associated with nasty side effects. Natural sleep aids are safe alternatives to sleeping pills. The following herbs are known as the natural sleep aids: Valerian, 5HTP (hydrotryptophan), L-Theanine, lavender tea, chamomile tea, and melatonin. [346]

CHERRIES are one of the few food sources of **melatonin,** a potent antioxidant produced naturally by the body's pineal gland, which helps regulate your biorhythm and natural sleep patterns. Scientists have found melatonin-rich Montmorency tart cherries contain more of this powerful antioxidant than what is normally produced by the body. Eating Montmorency cherries can be a natural way to boost your body's melatonin levels to hasten sleep and ease jet lag.

LEMON GRASS has a very high concentration of **citral,** a powerful antioxidant that has anti-tumor properties. It can help detoxification and aids in brain function. Lemongrass is also a sedative and has a relaxing effect on the brain, relieving stress and improving sleep patterns and insomnia.

PASSION FLOWER (*Passiflora inarnata*) has long been used to treat anxiety disorders. The extract of this flower has a mild sedative effect. Passionflower is believed to work by increasing the body's levels of a neurotransmitter called gamma amino butyric acid (GABA), which creates a relaxing effect by lowering the activity of some brain cells. The active compounds present in the extract include flavonoids such as **chrysin,** which mimic the action of benzodiazepine to produce a calming effect. Numerous studies have substantiated the claim that it encourages sleep and relieves nervous irritability. It also alleviates cramps that prevent deep and restful sleep.

VACATE

There are other methods for letting go of stress and toxic emotions beyond rest. One way is to get away from it all—vacate. A trip to a far-away destination is an ideal way to vacate, but don't think you always have to leave your hometown to take advantage of a good vacation. A nice afternoon in the **park** might be all you need.

The best vacations take place when you empty yourself of the inputs of everyday life. That's why a park is such a good place for a mini vacation; you can go there and get away from the hustle and bustle of life. All that's around you is **nature**, which should be a nice contrast to city living with its fast pace and many sources of frustration. But although vacating in a natural wonderland is an obvious way to clear your head, there are plenty of easy "vacations" you can take in your own home. Try fasting from some form of technology that usually consumes your day. **News fasts, TV fasts,** or **computer fasts** are all good ways to clear your mind of unnecessary negativity.

Another, less conventional idea for a vacation is to go on a **refrigerator fast.** We rely on refrigerators too much in this country, and they're really not good for you. Your body likes things to be hot; it's at a constant temperature of 98.6 degrees. Think about all the stress you put your body through when you give it cold foods. It has to fight to maintain its optimal temperature. A refrigerator fast will make you feel better because you will no longer force your body to work hard to maintain itself.

Clearing out your mind and body is important, but it's also crucial that you vacate your personal space. Eliminating unnecessary clutter from your closet, garage, and bedroom will help you feel better. **Decluttering** not only vacates your physical space, but it also helps clear out your mind. Another good way to clean your mind is to take deep breaths before you go to bed and immediately after waking up. Cleansing breaths will help get you ready for the day to come!

RECREATE

Get a life people! You've got to find something you love to do and take the time to do it on a regular basis. **Recreation** is another good way to overcome emotional issues. When you make yourself happy with something you enjoy, there's no way you can drown in your problems. So take up a new hobby, play with your kids or your kid-like friends, cook up a great meal, and make work fun again with inspiring office games.

This next piece of advice might sound silly, but it's something many people have problems doing. When you find a new hobby, make sure it is something you really enjoy doing. Don't take up a new pastime just because it's supposed to be fun—only do it if it actually is fun for you. For example, if all of your friends have gardening hobbies, you might think that gardening is a good way to spend your leisure time. If you like it, go for it. But if working in your yard is something you dread doing, find another activity. An enjoyable hobby will increase your energy levels, but if you get involved in something that you really don't like, your energy will be drained. Everyone likes different things, so take your time and find a pastime that you look forward to doing.

RELATE

We all need to relate to other people to be happy, but not just anyone will do. Have you ever been around people who are always **negative**? They never seem to see the bright side of life, and they always want help with their problems. How about unreliable people who will come to you when they need something but aren't around otherwise? These types of friends are toxic. There's no need to keep people who don't respect you and who don't help you in your life.

Everyone has a bad day now and then, and I'm not telling you to get rid of friends who are going through hard times and are depressed. You can't abandon your friends when they need you most. But if a person consistently makes you feel bad or guilty—and I'm talking over months and years—you owe it to yourself to create distance between you and the so-called friend. Give yourself an ultimatum: stop associating with these people unless they turn around. This goes for family members too, although you can't divorce yourself from your family forever.

Get rid of depressing friends and surround yourself with **happy people**. Find people who are uplifting and make an effort to get close to them. This isn't all about you, however. You need to become a happy person yourself. Be the person your friends call for advice; make yourself infective, so that after a long talk everyone feels better and wants more. If you want to make more friends, it starts with you. You can't sit around and wonder why people aren't approaching you. Make the first move! Reconnecting with old friends is another great way to relate and it's also a good remedy for boring routines. Call an old friend out of the blue; you'll definitely feel good afterward!

SELF TALK

As important as it is to have friends and relate to them, relating to yourself positively is perhaps even more crucial. Treat yourself just like you would treat your best friend. That means no negative self talk.[347] It can be easy to overanalyze your own behavior, but you have to try to avoid distorted thinking—don't be too hard on yourself.[348] Read over the list of **dos and don'ts** below to learn more ways to build a good relationship with yourself:

- **DON'T** criticize yourself for little things.
- **DON'T** set negative expectations.[349] This is setting yourself up for failure!
- **DON'T** tell yourself what you "should" be doing. Avoid "shoulds" altogether; it sets limits on how you are doing.[350]
- **DON'T** worry all the time.[351]
- **DON'T** become a victim of unhealthy guilt.[352]
- **DON'T** dwell on your mistakes.
- **DON'T** get too attached to your friends. Love them and care about them without getting enmeshed in their lives.[353]
- **DO** accept yourself for who you are.
- **DO** cultivate self compassion.
- **DO** love yourself.
- **DO** listen to your inner voice for guidance.[354]

SET GOALS

I recommend setting distinct goals in three areas of your life: **personal**, **professional**, and **relational**. **Personal goals** are all about you. They detail what you want to achieve with your body, your outlook, and your health. An example of a personal goal would be committing to losing 15 pounds by a specific date. **Professional goals,** on the other hand, have to do with how you perform on the job. You might want to get a raise within two years or go back to school by the time you're a certain age. Finally, **relational goals** are about how you interact with other people. For example, you might tell yourself that you'll go on more dates starting tomorrow. Or you may commit to spending a certain amount of time with your significant other each week.

The thing to remember about goals is they have to be **attainable.** You won't be motivated for long if your goals are out of reach. I recommend setting different levels of goals for yourself in each category. Try setting a **short-term** goal, **a long-term** goal, and a **lifetime** goal in each. A short-term goal should be reachable within a few months. A long-term goal may take more than a year to achieve. And a lifetime goal, obviously, is something you want to reach and maintain over your entire life. All three of these goals complement one another, so while you will have a vague, lifetime goal to work toward, you have more immediate, short-term goals that act as stepping stones to get there.

DAILY HOUR

I recommend you take an hour out of your busy life each day to rest, vacate, recreate, relate, and set goals. I call this the **"daily hour."** It will be your time of renewal and revival. It's your time to get ready for the next 23 hours that will make up your day. Do this every day and your life will be more meaningful, purposeful, and efficient. Most importantly, you will be able to overcome the darkness of the moon—those negative emotions and thoughts that cloud your subconscious mind.

SCHEDULE YOUR HEALTH

In the ideal schedule below, sleep takes up at least seven hours of each day. There's also an hour reserved for rest, vacating, relating, and goal setting. How do you compare to this ideal? Write in the times you sleep, rest, relate, vacate, and set goals on the empty chart below.

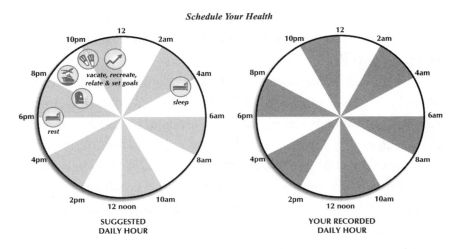

Schedule Your Health

SUGGESTED
DAILY HOUR

YOUR RECORDED
DAILY HOUR

REST, VACATE, RECREATE, RELATE, SET GOALS SCORING CHART

Circle the activities you do on a regular basis. Give yourself one point if more of your circles fall above the dotted line.

Rest, Vacate, Recreate, Relate, Set Goals Scoring Chart

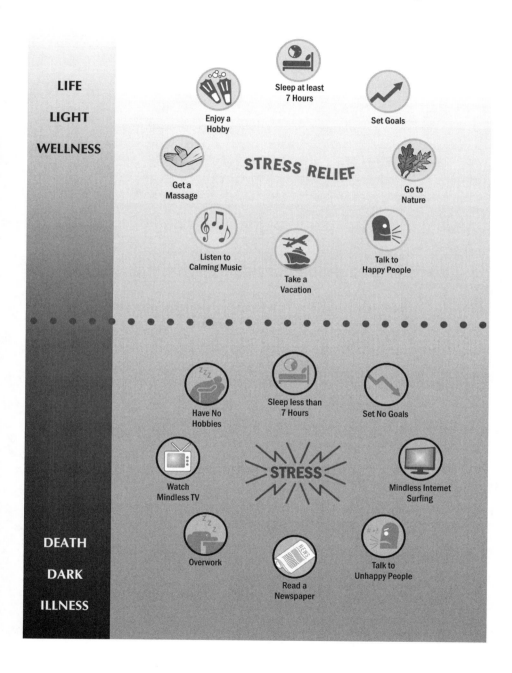

Chapter 9

THE 8TH SECRET:
SUN

"LOVE, ENJOY, APPRECIATE, FORGIVE"

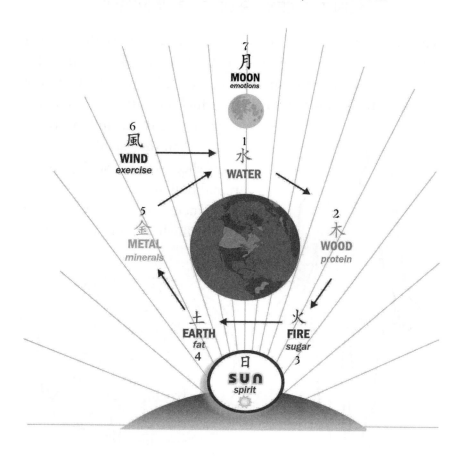

Our earth has no light of its own. Nor does the moon. It is the sun that gives light and life to the earth. Likewise, it is the spirit that gives us light and life. Just like plants need sunlight to survive and thrive, we need sunlight to live healthfully. Also, the spirit is the center of our being, just like the sun is the center of our solar system. When you bring the spiritual qualities of love, joy, appreciation, and forgiveness into your life, you will be able to chase away the darkness of stress. This is the true spiritual healing from God.

SUN, THE CENTER OF OUR UNIVERSE

The sun is the center of our solar system. It is the **driving force** behind the whole system, keeping the planets in orbit and warming our atmosphere so that life is possible. In a very real way, the sun is the power that fuels everything. Our sun is immense. It is 1.3 million times bigger than the earth![355] Because of its sheer size, the sun's gravitational pull makes the earth move at an incredible 67,000 miles per hour, which is more than 1,000

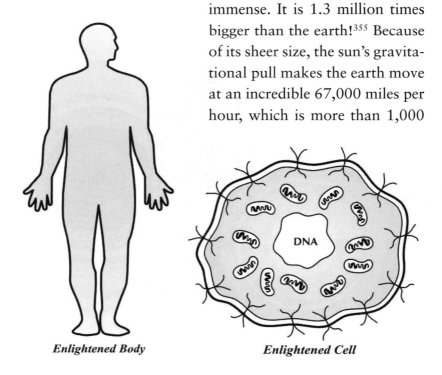

Enlightened Body   *Enlightened Cell*

times faster than the average speed on our freeways.[356] The sun's gravitational pull is enough to hold all the planets in their orbits. Even though the earth is 93 million miles away from the sun, the strength of our sun keeps us in place.[357]

Our sun is burning hot too. It is an unbelievable 27 million degrees Fahrenheit at its core![358] Even though we are so far away from the sun, it is hot and bright enough to burn our skin and our eyes. The sun helps our bodies function properly too. **Photons**, which are the smallest units of light, are responsible for communication between all of the cells in our bodies.

SUN, THE LIGHT, THE LIFE, AND THE SPIRIT

Physically, the sun is amazing. But it also has a spiritual dimension. We can think of the sun as a symbol that represents **light**, **life**, and **spirit**. Like the sun is the center of the solar system, the spirit is the center of our being. It controls our bodies and our minds. No matter how grim the night, the sun always returns and wipes out the darkness completely. Similarly, no matter how deep and terrible your stress or emotional wounds, spiritual qualities of love, appreciation, joy, and forgiveness can overcome them. In this chapter, you will learn about the power of the spirit and how it is manifested physically. The spirit—sunlight—is what truly sparks all the cells of your body to turn on your genes, which then replicate and thrive. Look at the previous pictures. As you can see, when you have the sun in your life, your body and cells are enlightened!

BENEFITS OF VITAMIN S

Since sunlight is so vital to us, I call it Vitamin S. We need a good deal of Vitamin S because it is what makes us have life.

Sunlight improves health and prevents illnesses. It gives us so many benefits! It can: [359]

THE BENEFITS OF SUNLIGHT	
SUNLIGHT IMPROVES...	**SUNLIGHT REDUCES...**
Elevate your mood and boost your mental performance	Prevent ovarian, prostate, breast, and many other cancers
Improve the function of your pancreas	Reduce your risk of melanoma, a deadly form of skin cancer
Increase insulin sensitivity and prevent diabetes	Prevent and treat bone diseases
Help you lose weight	Prevent depression and other mental disorders
Make you sleep better	Significantly lower high blood pressure
Give you more energy and stamina	Lower high blood sugar
Increase the white blood cells responsible for immunity	Decrease bad cholesterol in your blood

In addition to all the wonderful things listed above, light from the sun also prevents 17 different types of cancer.[360] It fends off unhealthy heart conditions.[361] It protects against diabetes.[362] It improves your immune system and your muscle strength[363]. It also enhances your sexual drive.[364]

I believe that sunlight is as important for our bodies as it is for **plants.** If plants don't get enough sunlight, the chlorophyll in their cells will not be activated, which means the plants won't be able to make their own food. Sunlight is everything to plants. It's also vital for our health, as you have seen by all the benefits it gives. Sunlight affects every cell and assists with every function in our bodies. In fact, it controls our every movement and rhythm.

USE SUNLIGHT AS MEDICINE

Nowadays, most Americans spend the majority of their time indoors. Only 10 percent of people work outside; most people work inside under artificial lights, travel inside cars to get anywhere, and use sunscreens when they are outdoors to block natural light.[365] This isn't good. There has been an increased frequency of disease as our exposure to sun has decreased. If you avoid being outside, you are living in darkness. Your eyes are your windows, through which light enters your body. Every two hours, your blood circulates through your eyes, and the nutrients in this blood are activated by the sunlight. If you aren't exposed to the sun, these nutrients aren't turned on.[366]

The sunlight that enters your body through your eyes stimulates your pineal gland, which is sometimes known as your third eye. When it is stimulated, the pineal gland produces **melatonin** and **serotonin**, two neurotransmitters that can improve your mental health. These neurotransmitters also signal the hypothalamus to activate your endocrine system, which produces all other hormones.[367] In short, sunlight gets your body working! Like oxygen and water, sunlight is one of the most important elements for your body, and medicine has been ignoring it for too long.

SUNLIGHT PRODUCES VITAMIN D

Your body produces vitamin D through a chain of reactions, which starts when sunlight hits your skin. Ultraviolet light makes contact with the pre-cholesterol on your skin to produce cholecalciferol, which is also known as vitamin D3. When vitamin D3 mixes with oxygen in your liver, it creates calcidiol, a biologically weak form of vitamin D. The vitamin is strengthened into its active form, called calcitrol, when it comes in contact with your kidneys and other tissues.[368] You can't make vitamin D without sunlight!

The primary job of vitamin D is to carry calcium into your cells. With **calcium**, vitamin D helps prevent cancer, inflammatory diseases, autoimmune diseases, and metabolic diseases.

Unfortunately, about 90 percent of the population lacks either sufficient vitamin D or calcium, which makes them more susceptible to all these problems.[369] In fact, your whole body depends on vitamin D to **turn on your genes** and direct the production of enzymes, proteins, hormones, neurotransmitters, and just about every organ you have![370]

It is absolutely necessary for everyone to have his or her vitamin D levels tested regularly. Get tested at least once each year to track your vitamin D levels and detect any health risks you may have. Ask your doctor for a **25-hyrdoxyvitamin D test,** which can be performed quickly in the office. Compare your results to the following optimal and normal levels of vitamin D.[371]

25-hydroxyvitamin D value	
OPTIMAL AMOUNT	NORMAL AMOUNT
50-60 ng/ml or 125-150 nmol/l	8-60 ng/ml or 20-150 nmol/l

REVERSE YOUR SHRINKING

You've probably heard that people shrink as they get older. This doesn't have to be the case with you! You shrink when you have **osteoporosis,** but sunlight can reverse the effects of this disease. Also, many older people suffer from **rickets,** a vitamin D deficiency disease that causes bowed legs and a hunched body. You can take all the calcium you want, but unless you get vitamin D from sunlight, your calcium will not get into your bones.[372]

RISKS OF VITAMIN D DEFICIENCY

You are more likely to be deficient in vitamin D if . . .

1. You live far away from the equator.
2. You are older. Compared to a 20-year-old person, elderly people get only 25 percent of vitamin D from the same amount of sunlight.
3. You have darker skin. Dark-skinned people need 10 to 50 times more sunlight to produce the same amount of vitamin D as a fair-skinned person.
4. You are obese.
5. You are not getting at least 15 to 20 minutes of sun three to five times each week.
6. You wear sunscreen with an SPF higher than eight. This decreases vitamin D production by 95 percent.
7. You have Crohn's disease, cystic fibrosis, celiac disease, or liver, hepatic, or kidney disease.
8. You take Phenytoin, Phenobarbital, or Rifampin. These drugs increase the breakdown of vitamin D in your liver.[373]

HOW TO GET ENOUGH VITAMIN D

For good health, you should get about 4,000 IU of vitamin D each day.[374] However, the FDA only recommends a daily dosage of 200 to 400 IU, which is less than 10 percent of what you really need. To get the optimal amount of vitamin D, you need to get more sun![375]

Getting this much sun each day can seem tough, especially if you have dark skin and need a lot. But if you involve yourself in more **outdoor activities**, you'll get enough sun the easy way. Start hiking, go on a picnic, play outdoor games, join a sports team, or just take a walk.[376] All of these things will make going outside and getting sunlight fun.

The sun can also improve your **sexual health**. Sitting naked in the sun is a sure way to increase testosterone levels and sexual vigor. For men, when the chest or back is exposed to sunlight, male hormones increase by 120 percent. When the genital area is exposed, the hormones can shoot up by 200 percent! Europeans, who are known for sunbathing naked, must have known about this for years![377]

If you find it impossible to spend time outside, you can get additional vitamin D by installing **full-spectrum lighting** inside.[378] You can buy this kind of lighting at most home-improvement stores, and it's easy to put up. Another thing you need to do to increase your levels of vitamin D is to supplement **cod liver oil** daily. One tablespoon of cod liver oil has 1200 to 1400 IU of the vitamin. Cod liver oil is an easy way to get plenty of vitamin D, so I recommend it above all else. But there are other foods that are high in vitamin D too. Look over the following table below to find out which foods are best for increasing your vitamin D levels.[379]

It's true that some foods, especially dairy products, are often fortified with vitamin D. However, the form of the vitamin included in these foods is chemically produced; it's not healthy for you, and you shouldn't rely on it for your vitamin D.[380]

FOODS HIGH IN VITAMIN D		
FOOD	SERVING SIZE	VITAMIN D AMOUNT (IU)
Cod Liver Oil	1 tablespoon	1360
Salmon (cooked)	3.5 oz.	360
Sardines (canned)	3.5 oz.	270
Tuna (canned)	3 oz.	200
Egg Yolk	1 yolk	25
Beef Liver (cooked)	3.5 oz.	15

TOXIC AND NATURAL SUNSCREENS

Most of the sunscreens available in stores contain toxic chemicals. They aren't good for you and should be avoided at all costs. If you buy sunscreen, check for these chemical names:

- Octyl-dimethyl-PABA (OD-PABA)
- Benzophenone-3 (Bp-3)
- Homosalate (HMS)
- Octyl-methoxycinnamate (OMC)
- 4-methyl-benzylidene camphor (4-MBC)[381]

The chemicals listed above are common in sunscreens, but they can all cause cancer cells to grow more rapidly than they would otherwise.[382] If you must wear sunscreen, use a natural product with **vitamins C and E** included. **Zinc oxide** is an excellent form of natural sunscreen, and I recommend using it on places that burn easily. Otherwise, cover yourself up to avoid exposing sensitive skin to strong sun rays. A sun umbrella, hat, and long sleeved pants and shirts are excellent ways to prevent sunburns without chemicals.

If you do get sunburned, use a water-based lotion with vitamins C and E to soothe your skin. Then, take an extra 400 IU dose of vitamin E before you go to bed to help repair any damage.[383]

LOVE

As we have seen, the physical sun is important for our health. However, the spiritual center that is represented by the figure of the sun is perhaps even more crucial in our lives. We can compare the sun to the awesome power of God.

God shows His love through you. He loves to express Himself as harmony, peace, beauty, joy, and abundance. This is God's love and the tendency of every life.[384] It is what St. Paul said is the true meaning of love: "Love is patient, love is kind. It does not envy, it does not boast, it is not proud. It is not rude, it is not self-seeking, it is not easily angered, it keeps no record of wrongs. Love does not delight in evil but rejoices with the truth. It always protects, always trusts, always hopes, always perseveres."[385] St. Paul could not express love in just a few words. Instead, he spent a whole chapter describing it.

In the Bible, one of the teachers of the law asks Jesus about the most important commandments. Jesus replies, "**Love the Lord your God** with all your heart, and with all your soul, and will all your mind, and with all your strength. The second is this: **Love your neighbors** as yourself."[386] As Jesus said, love is the most important thing you can do. You need to use everything you have physically, mentally, emotionally, and spiritually to love God. When this happens, then you are capable of loving other people.

When you truly experience the love of God, you will open the eyes of love in your body and soul. I have experienced this myself and will share my personal story in Chapter 11. Since we have no light of our own, we are not capable of loving others perpetually without God. With God's help, you can love others as yourself, which means that you will not be selfish anymore. "You" and "I" will finally be "we." This is how we truly love others—with God. This is also how to truly solve all the problems of relationships.

LOVE TALK

One of the most profound books about love is called *The Five Love Languages* by Dr. Gary Chapman. In his book, Dr.

Chapman talks about different love languages that people use to communicate. We all have one language that we understand the most, and we feel loved when we receive messages in our primary language. The five love languages are: words of affirmation, quality time, gifts, acts of service, and physical touch.[387]

My primary love language is acts of service, which means I feel most loved when people do things for me. When my wife cooks, cleans, does my laundry, and prepares seminar slides for me, I feel loved. My wife, on the other hand, feels most loved by my physical touch. When I kiss her, caress her, and hug her, she feels the most love. She especially likes when I give her massages, so I try to give her a massage every night before we go to bed. For many years before I read Dr. Chapman's book, I tried to express my love for my wife through my **own love language,** acts of service. I tried to do things for her, but she did not feel any love from these things. We all try to express our love through our own language, but the receiver may not understand our language. When you and your partner speak two different love languages, you could have some serious problems with miscommunication.

Take the following test to find out **your own love language.** Then ask your spouse or partner to take the test too. That way, you'll understand what makes you feel loved and how you can share your love with your partner. If you can learn to speak the other person's love language, your relationship will literally transform. For this test, simply insert the name of your spouse, significant other, or another companion into the blank spaces. Then, choose what you think is the best answer to each question. At the end of the test, tally the total number of each letter you have to determine your love language.[388]

S. DON KIM

1. Sweet love notes from _____ make me feel good. . . . . .A

   I love _____'s hugs. . . . . E

2. I like to be alone with _____. . . . . .B

   I feel loved when _____ washes my car. . . . . .D

3. Receiving special gifts from _____ makes me happy. C

   I enjoy long trips with _____. . . . . .B

4. I feel loved when _____ helps me with the laundry. . . . . .D

   I like it when _____ touches me. . . . . E

5. I feel loved when _____ puts his/her arm around me. . . . . E

   I know _____ loves me because he/she surprises
   me with gifts. C

6. I like going most anywhere with _____. . . . . .B

   I like to hold _____'s hand. . . . . E

7. I value the gifts _____ gives to me. C

   I love to hear _____ say that he/she loves me. . . . . A

8. I like for _____ to sit close to me. . . . . E

   _____ tells me I look good, and I like that. . . . . A

9. Spending time with _____ makes me happy. . . . . B

   Even the smallest gift from _____ is important to me. C

10. I feel loved when _____ tells me he/she is proud of me. . . . . . A

    When _____ cleans up after a meal, I know that
    he/she loves me. . . . . .D

11. No matter what we do, I love doing things with _____. . . . . . .B

    Supportive comments from _____ make me feel good. . . . . . .A

12. Little things _____ does for me mean more

    to me than words. . . . . .D

    I love to hug _____. . . . . E

13. _____'s praise means a lot to me. . . . . .A

    It means a lot to me that _____ gives me gifts I really like. C

14. Just being around _____ makes me feel good. . . . . B

    I love when _____ gives me a massage. . . . . E

15. _____'s reactions to my accomplishments are so encouraging. . . . . A

It means a lot when _____ helps with something I know he/she hates. . . . . D

16. I never get tired of _____'s kisses. . . . . E

I love that _____ shows real interest in things I like to do. . . . . B

17. I can count on _____ to help me with projects. . . . . D

I still get excited when opening a gift from _____. C

18. I love for _____ to compliment my appearance. . . . . A

I love that _____ listens to me and respects my ideas. . . . . B

19. I can't help but touch _____ when he/she is close by. . . . . E

_____ sometimes runs errands for me, and I appreciate that. . . . . D

20. _____ deserves an award for all the things he/she does to help me. . . . . D

I'm sometimes amazed at how thoughtful _____'s gifts to me are. C

21. I love having _____'s undivided attention. . . . . B

I love that _____ helps me clean the house. . . . . D

22. I look forward to seeing what _____ gives me for my birthday. C

I never tire of hearing _____ tell me that I am important to him/her. . . . . A

23. _____ lets me know he/she loves me by giving me gifts. C

_____ shows his/her love by helping me without me having to ask. . . . . D

24. _____ doesn't interrupt me when I'm talking, and I like that. . . . . B

I never get tired of receiving gifts from _____. C

25. _____ is good about asking me how he/she can help when I'm tired. . . . . D

It doesn't matter where we go, I just like going places with _____. C

26. I love cuddling with _____. . . . . E

    I love surprise gifts from _____. C

27. _____'s encouraging words give me confidence. . . . . A

    I love to watch movies with _____. . . . . B

28. I couldn't ask for any better gifts than the
    ones _____ gives me. C

    I love it that _____ can't keep his/her hands off me. . . . . E

29. It means a lot to me when _____ helps me
    despite being busy. . . . . D

    It makes me feel good when _____ tells me he/she
    appreciates me. . . . . A

30. I love hugging and kissing _____ after we've been apart
    for a while. . . . . E

    I love hearing _____ tell me that he/she missed me. . . . . A

Total A:_____ B:_____ C:_____ D:_____ E: _____

A = Words of Affirmation;

B = Quality time;

C = Receiving gifts;

D = Acts of service;

E = Physical touch.

WAYS TO EXPRESS LOVE

I feel God's love through my wife everyday. When I leave home every morning, my wife comes all the way to the street to wave goodbye. I live on the top of the hill and as I leave her, she waves her arms until I can't see her anymore through my rearview mirror. She says, "Have a great day" before I get into my car. I think this kind of love is exactly what we need to get through our stressful days. We need to give out this kind of love so that we can receive it back. If you don't have love like this, you should check to see if you are giving your family love. If not, start making an effort to love everyone a little bit harder. You'll see that your love will get you more love in return.

There are many ways you can express your love, and some are more personal than others. For your spouse or significant other, you can write **love letters, send flowers,** or **cook** a delicious meal. To show your family and friends how much you love them, give them **hugs** or offer to help out the next time they face a big project. Also, don't forget to show the world how much you love being alive and appreciate all human life. **Volunteer** to help other people if you can.

LOVE OF LORTH: ANT KINGDOM STORY

Once upon a time, there was Lorth. He had the power to create anything he loved. He so loved the ants that he created them out of his pure love. He created the ant kingdom for the ants because he wanted to have an intimate relationship with the ants. He wanted the ants to love one another and to live in harmony with other ants as they were designed to be. Unfortunately, the ants started to ignore Lorth and killed one another. Lorth sent many of his messengers who spoke the ants' language to the ant kingdom. These messengers told the ants to turn to Lorth and love the other ants. The messengers, who were named Isaiath, Jeremiath, Zechariath, and many others, were bitten and killed by the ants. They wouldn't listen.

Finally, Lorth became frustrated with his creations and sent Jesuth, his only son. Jesuth told the ants about Lorth's love for them. When the ants did not listen, Lorth had Jesuth die for the ants to show the unconditional love of Lorth for the ants. Through his life and death as an ant, Jesuth showed that only through him could the ants enter the kingdom of Lorth and have an intimate relationship with Him who created them. This is the most tragic yet victorious love story of all time.

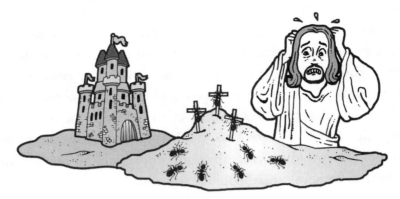

Love of Lorth: Ant Kingdom Story

Obviously, this story is an allusion to the love that God, our creator, has for us. You can see this in the illustration. God loves us so much that he sent his only son, Jesus, to redeem us. The ant story was inspired by the fact that ants and humans are the only animals that knowingly kill their own race. Last century, we killed about 260 million people in war. Why won't we listen to God's commandment and love one another?

ENJOY

Enjoy literally means joy that comes from within. Cursory joy can come from the external world of our material possessions, achievements, and acquired positions. But true and lasting joy only comes from the **unseen world** within us. There are three different ways you can bring joy instantly. The first is the expectation of an event, people, or other things. The second way is through the actual event, when your expectation comes true. And the third way to bring joy is in remembering these past events.[389] To harness these ways of bringing joy, try making lists of special places, people, pets, animals, activities, peak experiences, religious experiences, textures, scents, tastes, sounds, and colors.[390] Read over your list whenever you need a boost of pure joy.

Practice your inner smile, which is that warm, caring, and watchful sensation that is most easily started in your heart. An **inner smile** of joy will spread throughout your whole body.[391] There is science behind why you feel so good when you smile. Smiling eyes produce a continuous flow of endorphins.[392] And when you smile, you open yourself up to the experience of joy. That's because to find joy, you must make yourself relaxed, safe, and confident.[393]

HAPPINESS IS A HABIT

When I give seminars, I usually take a moment and ask the audience to try to be happy. Immediately after I say this, the mood of the crowd changes; the room becomes full of joy and pleasant energy. Using the feeling in the room as an example, I tell the audience they have a choice to be happy or unhappy during every moment of their lives. For most people, however, it is difficult to choose happiness. Unfortunately, your body, which is like the earth, has no light of its own. That's why it's easier and more comfortable for you to be in the darkness, the unhappiness. Happiness takes hard work. It requires you to **get in the habit** of reflecting on all of our decisions, asking ourselves, "Will this make me happy or unhappy?"

Our biggest problem in achieving happiness is our inability to be satisfied. We have an insatiable desire to do more and have more things.[394] This **dissatisfaction** with the status quo allows us to accomplish more, but it also makes us unhappy.[395] Also, when there is a difference between what we want and what we get, we become unhappy, thus adding to our inability to be satisfied.[396] We tend to focus on the negatives of what we don't have rather than the positives of what we do have.[397]

HOW TO BE HAPPY

You will be happy when you do the following things:
- Find **meaning** and **purpose** in your life.[398]
- Don't lose sight of your **goals**.[399]
- Find **positive** aspects of every situation, even the negative ones.[400]
- Seek to do **good** no matter what.[401]
- Find **good people** and keep them around.[402]

LAUGHTER IS THE BEST MEDICINE

Let me tell you a true story about the power of laughter. When Norman Cousins came back from a trip to China, he became severely ill. He was diagnosed with ankylosing spondylitis, a disease in which the spine disintegrates. He was in so much pain that he couldn't sleep at all. By coincidence, at the time of his diagnosis, he was studying the effects of **endorphins** on pain, so he decided to do a test on himself. Cousins sat up and watched funny videos. He laughed all night. To his amazement, he was able to sleep for one hour after an hour of belly laughs. In time, he was laughing so hard that he got kicked out of the hospital!

Cousins literally laughed his way back to health, and he told the whole world about his laughter therapy and its effects on healing. Through laughter, Cousins was completely healed. He wrote a bestselling book, *Anatomy of an Illness*, and traveled the world sharing his amazing story. As Cousins learned, when you laugh, your body produces powerful endorphins that can cure almost any disease known to mankind. Unfortunately, we do not use this wonderful free medicine often enough. In fact, a recent survey found that 4-year-old children laugh an average of 400 times per day; comparatively, 50-year-olds only laugh three times per day! This lack of laughter is a huge epidemic, and it's one that has terrible health consequences.

ENDORPHINS, THE ELIXIR OF LIFE

When they were first discovered, endorphins amazed scientists. They still do. The name "endorphins" comes from "**endogenous morphine**" because the substances were originally thought to be morphine that is produced in the body.[403] Now we know that endorphins are neuropeptides, chemicals which carry information around the body. Interestingly, endorphins are chemically similar to opium and morphine. So far, 20 different types of endorphins have been discovered.[404]

Previously, we thought that only the brain produced endorphins, but now we know that they come from all over the body. For example, your adrenal glands produce some types of endorphins.[405] Endorphins are some of the most helpful and most powerful drugs available to us—they are **200 times** more powerful than morphine and aren't dangerous. They can create physical pleasure and kill pain; work towards the healing of wounded and diseased tissues; boost the immune system; create physical feelings of wellbeing, which can foster emotional and mental wellbeing; and create euphoria and bliss states.[406] Endorphins also activate natural killer (NK) cells, which can kill cancer cells.

Amazingly, you can trigger the production of endorphins at will.[407] All you have to do is realize the beauty of your life. Feel satisfaction in being alive and ponder the connection between yourself, the universe, and your creator. Then, you will let the endorphins flood in. Changing your perception of your surroundings can also help trigger endorphins.[408] It's like training yourself to be happy. Train yourself to see the world as an exciting, pleasurable place and your endorphins will flow. It is not necessary to wait for external sources to release endorphins; just change your **internal perception** to reap the rewards.

ENDORPHIN ADDICTIONS

For most people, endorphins are something of a miracle drug. But some people experience a **negative side** to endorphins—addiction. People with **anorexia nervosa** have a version of endorphin addiction. They are addicted to self starvation; they release endorphins when they lose weight and always want to continue the euphoria, so they keep starving. Non-eating and weight loss promotes a sense of well being for anorexics because their moods are improved by endorphins.[409] Other endorphin addicts tend to exercise to the point of physical trauma and deterioration of health.[410] I know some runners and other athletes who keep running to the point of physical breakdown. This is from pure addiction, and it's very dangerous to their health.

APPRECIATE

A lot of times, we take people and things in our lives for granted. For example, if you're married, you probably forget about all that your spouse does for you at times. Similarly, many of us don't take the time to reflect on how lucky we are to be alive and living in a wealthy country. Even if you can barely make ends meet, you're better off than many homeless, destitute people in this world. Do you ever take the time to thank God for your blessings? If you're like most people, you don't do it enough. That's where appreciation comes in.

Appreciation means being thankful. It's closely linked to love. Like love, appreciation requires that you reach out to other people. Stop for a second and think about the people in your life you should appreciate. Write thank-you letters to these people—your parents, friends, coworkers, spouse, neighbors, etc. Although sharing your thankful feelings is best, it's okay if you don't want to actually mail these letters. Just writing about your appreciation will be enough to help you realize your many blessings. Take the time to write a **thank-you letter** to God, too. He is the source of your happiness, and it's beneficial to reflect on His goodness.

Another way you can help yourself appreciate your many gifts is to create a **thank-you box**. Collect reminders of all the things that you are thankful for and put them in your box. For example, if your neighbor regularly helps you around the house, you might want to put a photo of him in your thank-you box. At the end of the year or perhaps on Thanksgiving, go through your collection in your box and remember all that you have to be thankful for. You came into this world with nothing; appreciate all that you now have.

Appreciation will not only help you, but it will also help those you care about. Just **showing** your love and appreciation will make you and your loved ones healthier. Dr. Masuru Emoto proved this to be so. He gave information to water by either talking to it or writing words on the outside of water-filled glasses. Then, he froze the water to -20 degrees Celsius, or -4 degrees Fahrenheit, for three hours. After the three hours, Dr. Emoto allowed the ice to melt. He took pictures of the melting ice crystals and was shocked by the results. The crystals were beautiful when they were exposed to positive words and classical music, but they were deformed when exposed to harsh language. The most beautiful crystals of all were those exposed to the words **"love and gratitude."**[411] This is proof that what we don't see is infinitely more powerful than what we do see. Look at the following illustration to see how beautiful the crystal is. Your appreciation can work miracles. Compare that to bad words like "you, idiot"

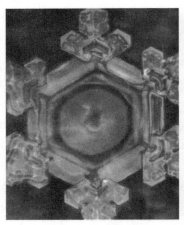 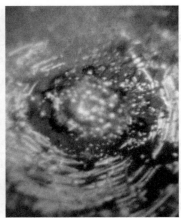

"Thank You"   *"You Idiot!"*

FORGIVE

FORGIVING IS FREEDOM. When you forgive, you free yourself from self-inflicted bondage. In other words, you must forgive others to help yourself. Most of the time, when you struggle about someone who hurt you, the other person doesn't even realize that you are upset with them. You are not hurting anyone but yourself when you refuse to offer forgiveness.

Forgiveness is the hardest part of this secret for many people. It's hard to let go of past offenses from other people, but it's even harder to forgive ourselves for our mistakes and failures. The truth is, many of us like holding grudges and not forgiving. However, nothing good comes from resentment; it only leads to anger, selfishness, and poor health. Refusing to forgive is just like subjecting your body to unnecessary stress. You release negative hormones and get fat! So let go of your grudges. Forgive other people and yourself and you'll experience a healthy flow of endorphins.

There are four levels of giving, and forgiving is the most complete kind of gift. These levels are:

1. NOT GIVING BACK. Some people are selfish, and when you give, they don't reciprocate.

2. GIVING BACK. Most people do this. When you give something, they give something back.

3. GIVING. This is when endorphins start flowing in your body. You are giving without expecting anything in return. You are just giving out of the goodness of your heart.

4. FOR-GIVING. This is the highest level of giving. The other person has done something terrible to you and your instinct is to not give at all. But you give anyway, despite the other person's actions. When you do this, healing juices are flowing!

EVERLENE'S TESTIMONY

Before I met Dr. Kim, I was really angry. I was angry at my doctors and angry at my family. My anger started when I was a child. I was the youngest of 10 children. My family all had dark skin, but I came out light. Everyone made fun of me for that, and I took it personally. Also, I injured my back working as a schoolteacher. I saw two doctors who belittled me. They didn't really care about me and disrespected me every time I saw them. I was angry with them too. I was very resentful and couldn't forgive my family or the doctors. Because of my back pain, I couldn't walk without crutches or a walker for seven years.

I saw Dr. Kim because the arch in my foot had collapsed. I told him about my problems, and he asked me to pray with him about it. He told me my body could heal if I could love and forgive. So I prayed. I said, "I want to be able to forgive. I want to be rid of my anger." Dr. Kim prayed with me and believed with me. That day, I was just at the bottom. But I truly felt that I wanted to forgive. When I offered forgiveness to my family and my doctors, I felt something hot in my back.

I didn't know I was healed in the office that day. However, the next morning, I could walk again without crutches. It was a miracle! I was healed spiritually, and the physical healing followed. That's how my miracle worked. I still have my same body. And it still hurts if I over work it. But in spite of the pain, I can function now. I can forgive now too, and I believe my forgiveness is what cured me.

POWER OF PRAYER

Two-thirds of Americans report that they pray daily. Billions of people in most cultures, races, and religions pray daily. Prayer is the universal means by which human beings ask God for help.[412] However, about 90 percent of Americans would rather die than try healing prayer, the kind of prayer that is meant to bring miracles. Most of the other 10 percent of Americans see healing prayer as something they would do only as a last resort after conventional and alternative medicine.[413] This is unfortunate.

THOUGHTS ARE THINGS. Matter can be controlled and directed by thought, and that thought is a form of energy.[414] This life energy can be harnessed by prayer and used to heal.[415] We are all creators, and we are constantly creating good and bad things through the use or misuse of our power. We create by our thoughts, and every thought is prayer. If we visualize it and believe it, it will come about.[416]

Prayer gives **healing energy**. The Chinese call it "chi." Indians call it "prana," "the essence of life." Obviously, prayer is important all over the world. Why don't people believe in its healing potential? Because belief in prayer hinges on faith. Dr. Olga Worrall, a renowned spiritual healer, put it best when she said, "How can anything like spiritual healing be proven conclusively in a material way?" I agree with her completely.

Here is an example of how Dr. Emoto's water crystals changed after prayer. Here is proof that prayer really works.

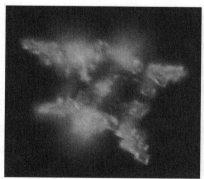
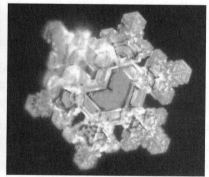

Before Prayer　　　　　　　*After Prayer*

EFFECTIVE PRAYER

Many prayers are not answered because they are not done properly. Prayer should never recite or concentrate on a problem. Instead, it should always describe or visualize the desired condition of perfect health.[417] In other words, you should visualize that your illness or problems have **already healed** for the best results.

There are four ways that prayers get answered:[418]

1. DIRECT CONTACT. When a sick person is physically touched.
2. DISTANT NO CONTACT. Energy that is present everywhere flows into the sick person.
3. POWER OF SUGGESTION. This happens when a thought can be firmly implanted in the mind of the sick person.
4. ATTUNEMENT. Raising the vibration of a sick person and bringing the person to a state that enables them to receive healing energy.

All four of these prayer styles will give results, but they all require one, underlying thing: **loving concern.** You need **love,** an **intention** to heal, and **faith** if you hope to heal through prayers.[419]

MY PERSONAL EXPERIENCE IN HEALING PRAYERS

I have heard of and seen many people who have been healed of supposedly incurable diseases, like malignant end-stage cancers, through the power of healing prayers. I have been praying for my patients' healing on my own for many years. It was not until about three years ago that I began offering healing prayers for my patients when they came to see me in my office. So far, I have had three of my patients heal miraculously from their diseases. I was shocked when it first happened and wanted to know more about it. I went to several weekend retreats known for spiritual healings to learn more.

Last year at Big Bear Mountain, I attended a healing seminar. I prayed the whole weekend to receive the ability to channel power and heal my patients. At one point in the weekend, we had a foot-washing ceremony. Right before it began, a message came to my heart. I started to cry. I cried for almost an hour. I couldn't stop. The message I had received was, "If you have the compassion, humility, and love to stoop down and wash these people's feet, then I will give you the ability to channel my healing power through you." From that moment on, I realized that all of us have this means to be conduits of God's healing power. We just need to cultivate **compassion, humility,** and **love** to use this gift.

SPIRITUAL HEALING

In the Old Testament of the Bible, the state of the nation's physical health was a reflection of its **spiritual condition.**[420] Almost every illness recorded in the Old Testament was a result of sin and disobedience.[421] In the New Testament, sickness is seen as an extension and effect of sin and is therefore evil in origin, representing the kingdom of Satan.[422] In other words, **healing is what God wants.** Of the 1257 verses in the Gospels, 484 verses, or 38.5 percent, are devoted to describing 41 instances of Jesus' healing ministries.[423]

Spiritual healing is far greater than the greatest physical healing because it is a new birth experience.[424] When you receive God's love and grace, you will be born again to become a new person. This is the true essence of spiritual healing. If you are completely mastered by the will of God, you will not be defeated by sickness, mental strain, disappointment, or temptation.[425] Health is the state of being in spiritual healing.

AREAS OF SPIRITUAL HEALING

We all need spiritual healing in four areas:

1. IN OUR SPIRITS. You need to restore your relationship with God, who designed you and created you.[426]

2. PAST EMOTIONAL HURTS. You need to heal from hurtful memories and damaged emotions from your past.[427]

3. MENTAL AND PSYCHOLOGICAL ILLNESSES. You need to heal from demonic and satanic forces that possess you through spiritual warfare.[428]

4. DYING AND DEATH. You need comforting and strengthening when you are dying.

MY OWN SPIRITUAL HEALING

I wanted to be a doctor all my life. I wanted to be in a profession where I could heal people from their physical sufferings. All throughout my medical training, I learned to heal my patients of their physical ailments only. At that time, I never realized that I would ever be talking about spiritual healing, not to mention emotional healing. Just as I started this chapter with the sun, which represents the light, the life, and the spirit, so do I want to end this chapter with the importance of receiving the light, the life, and the spirit during every waking moment of your life.

Without the presence of the spirit in your life, you will have **no lasting power**. Without getting enough love, joy, gratitude, and forgiveness, your health will suffer greatly. Unfortunately, our current healthcare system does not address these issues enough. This is what I believe is the biggest problem of our health crisis. After all, God wants to heal the whole person, not just his or her specific health conditions.[429] Since we are so focused on physical healing—and occasionally on emotional healing—we are not getting healed in the deepest part of who we are.

You need to receive the light. You need to receive **God's love.** You need to receive God's healing power every waking moment of your life to be healthy. Since you are dark and don't have any light of your own, it is crucial that you receive the light to spark all of your cells to function properly. It is time to take off the dark blanket that is covering every cell in your body. Let the light of God's spirit shine upon you completely! I will share with you how God's love and power came into my heart in Chapter 11.

SCHEDULE YOUR HEALTH

Look at the suggested activities for your spiritual activities on the chart to the left. Now, write in the activities that you do to keep your spirit healthy.

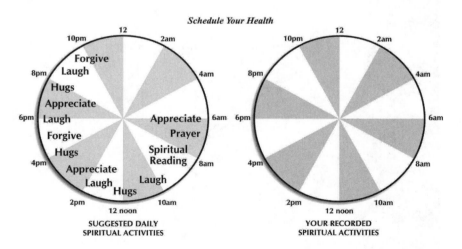

Schedule Your Health

SUGGESTED DAILY
SPIRITUAL ACTIVITIES

YOUR RECORDED
SPIRITUAL ACTIVITIES

SPIRITUAL WELLNESS SCORING CHART

Look at the following chart. Circle the spiritual activities you do on a regular basis. Give yourself one point if more of your circles fall above the dotted line.

Rest, Vacate, Recreate, Relate, Set Goals Scoring Chart

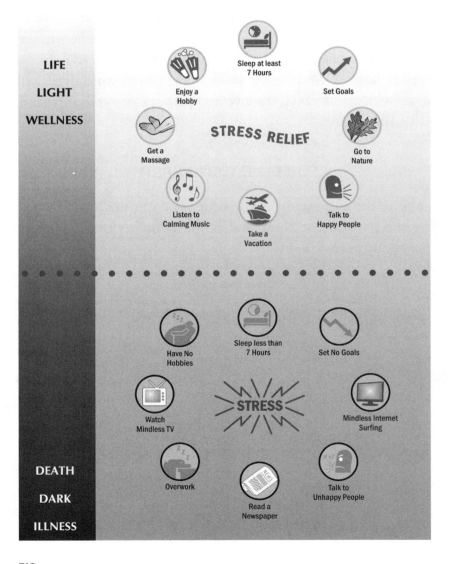

Chapter 10

METABOLISM AND WEIGHT LOSS

I want to take a few pages to summarize what we've learned so far in this book and tell you how it applies to your metabolism. Understanding your metabolism will help you lose weight, and since many people come to my seminars with weight loss as one of their main goals, I think it is important to address this issue.

So far, you've learned that your body has to turn like the earth. I liken this movement to your metabolism. When the earth turns and creates wind, that is, when you exercise, you start increasing your metabolism. When the moon rotates around the earth, that is, when you pay attention to your emotions, the pull of the moon can hinder or enhance the rotation of the earth, hence changing your metabolism. But what really makes the earth rotate—and your metabolism kick in gear—is the sun. By bringing in the light and the spiritual aspect of who you are, you will be able to optimize your metabolic function. When you understand the intricate workings of the eight elements of health that you have learned so far, you will be able to maximize your health.

METABOLISM AND WEIGHT LOSS

Your **metabolism** is the sum total of all the chemical reactions in your body plus everything you think, feel, and believe.[430] In other words, your metabolism is how your body does what it needs to do; the cells in your body are constantly destroyed or damaged by the wear and tear of living, and each day your metabolism repairs and regenerates these cells. Your metabolism is also how your body creates new hormones, enzymes, neurotransmitters, and other cellular chemicals to help you perform your daily tasks. There are two sides to your metabolism: the part that **uses up** energy and cells and the part that **rebuilds.**[431]

Your metabolism is equivalent to the **speed** at which the previous eight elements of health move in synchronicity. Just like the earth constantly turns on its axis and moves around the sun, so your metabolism needs to be in constant motion. When your metabolism is at its optimal speed and maintains regular movement, you will be able to eliminate toxins and extra weight naturally. As I have discussed throughout this entire book, when you change your lifestyle to increase and optimize your metabolism, you will lose all the weight you want, maintain your optimal weight, and get healthy.

After looking at many different medical approaches from many parts of the world, I discovered that there are many different metabolic types. Chinese medicine devised Yin and Yang energetic types along with 5 elemental types of earth that are discussed in this book. Ayurvetic medicine from India divided bodily constitution into 3 different types. My native country

Korea started with 4 metabolic types and now uses 8 metabolic types. They determine which foods should be eaten and which foods to avoid. Egyptians believe in 7 organ systems and eat according to these.

It is not the purpose of this book to go into details of these metabolic types. However, I believe that metabolic typing is very important because one size just does not fit all! I feel that understanding individual differences is crucial in taking control of your health more precisely. I will discuss this topic in upcoming books.

METABOLISM AND DETOXIFICATION LIFESTYLE

With any program, your goal should never simply be to lose weight. Instead, weight loss should be a natural result of **lifestyle changes**. You need to get healthy before you shed pounds. Once your metabolism normalizes to the rhythmic movement of your life, it will naturally remove your excess fats, which are storage units for unhealthy toxins. After your metabolism gets adjusted to your healthy lifestyle, there will be no reason for you to have stored fat. Your body won't be preparing for disaster any more.

Weight loss should not be a stressful way of living; instead it should be healthful and happy way of life. The natural, metabolism-driven way to lose weight is what I call the **detoxification lifestyle**. If you're like most people, the way you live now is very toxic. There's no way for you to avoid absorbing many of the toxins you come into contact with. However, if you live the detoxification lifestyle, you should be able to get rid of all the toxins that are coming into you daily. As you increase your metabolism to its optimal level, you will be able to eliminate the toxins from your body more efficiently.

METABOLISM AND EATING HABITS

For your metabolism to function at its best, you need to **super hydrate**. And this super hydrating needs to start first thing in the morning. You have been dehydrated from not drinking any fluid for the seven to nine hours you were asleep. As soon as you wake up, you need to drink a glass of water with a tablespoon of unrefined (natural) salt. Again, some people can't tolerate this at first, so start with a smaller amount and work up to one tablespoon. After this first glass of water, you need to drink half of your body weight in fluid ounces over the course of the day. Just drinking this recommended amount of water will speed up your metabolism tremendously.

Another important thing you must do in the morning is **eat**. Literally, you need to break your fast from the night with **long, robust, sit-down breakfast**. Numerous studies show that thin, healthy people eat breakfast every morning. The principles of chrononutrition—or eating at appropriate times—say that you have all the necessary enzymes for optimal digestion available in the morning, so you can and should have a feast for breakfast. I believe that skipping breakfast or eating a bad first meal is the single biggest health risk in this country. Sugar-rich breakfast foods such as pancakes, muffins, cereals, donuts, bagels, and other American favorites produce insulin, which is a neurotransmitter that tells the brain to eat more sugar all day long. You set your tone for the rest of the day with what you eat for breakfast. For the best health and the best metabolism, you need a **protein-rich breakfast** with plenty of good **fruits** and **vegetables**.

Lunch should be a **strong and relaxed meal**. At lunchtime, your body still has enough of the three enzymes needed for digestion: lipase, protease, and amylase. With these enzymes, you can break down a large amount of food, so you shouldn't be afraid to eat a big meal. You still have another half day to work, so you need to eat well. Many people eat lunch sitting at their desks or under stress—this is not good! You need to relax more while eating for the best results.

Contrary to what you might think and practice, **dinner** should be your smallest meal of the day because in the evening, you no longer need much fuel. Dinner should be **light and social.** During dinnertime, your body virtually stops producing any digestive enzymes. Therefore, a huge meal would just sit in your stomach and not get digested. This is devastating and it's why many people are overweight—they eat too much at night!

I also recommend you take **supplements** during your meals. **Digestive enzymes** are especially important to supplement; the excess processing and cooking of food will kill all the natural digestive enzymes available. This is why millions of people are taking antacids every day; they don't have any way to digest their food. Also add **probiotics** to enhance digestion and boost your immune system. **Snacks** between meals are also important if you want to increase your metabolism. If you eat small amounts of **fruits, vegetables, nuts, and seeds** throughout the day, your metabolism will be enhanced greatly. If you wait until you get hungry to eat, you will always overeat and become fat.

Eating under stress will slow down your metabolism. Stress includes eating too fast, not chewing enough, fostering guilt about your food, and not breathing while eating. All of these things will cause a decrease of nutrient absorption and an increase in your cholesterol levels, triglyceride levels, nutrient excretions from your body, salt retention, and many more negative effects.[432] Getting control of your breathing is particularly important for improving your metabolism. Taking three **deep breaths** before each meal can increase oxygenation, so you will be able to burn more calories.[433]

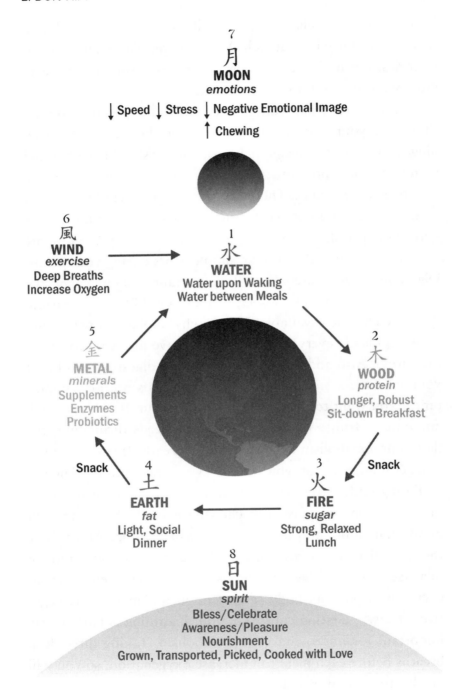

Practicing a **spiritual way of eating** can enhance your metabolism. So **bless** your food and the people who prepared it for you. Additionally, **celebrating** the food and meal will also increase your metabolism. Think about French people, who are known to truly celebrate their meals. Even though they consume just as much as food as Americans, French people don't get fat because they take their time and enjoy eating.[434] The next time you have a meal, try to experience the food, touch it, savor it, notice it, smell it, and ponder its color. When you feel pleasure in your food, your endorphins kick in to pump up your metabolic rate.[435]

RULE OF HANDS, RULE OF THUMBS.

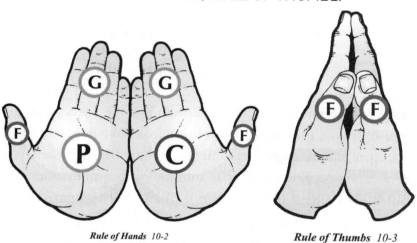

Rule of Hands 10-2　　　　　*Rule of Thumbs 10-3*

You are probably used to seeing the food pyramid, the government-issued guide to how you should eat. But the food pyramid is confusing because it is vague: it doesn't tell you how big a serving is! Instead of the food pyramid, I have devised an easy to way to remember how much to eat from each food group.

THE RULE OF HANDS states that you need to eat as much as both of your hands three times a day. For each meal, have the food on your plate equal the size and thickness of your hands. As you can see in the picture, green vegetables (G) should fill up the size of both hands' fingers at each meal. Make one of your palms equal to your protein (P) and the other the same size as your carbohydrates (C). THE RULE OF THUMBS means that you need to consume thumb-sized quantities of good fat (F) three times each day to keep healthy. Make your fat intake at each meal equivalent to the size of both thumbs. If you truly want to get healthy and lose weight, you should eat more for breakfast and less for dinner. I propose you eat three hands worth of food for breakfast, two for lunch, and one for dinner.

NUTRIENTS VS. NOURISHMENT

Yes, there is a difference between nutrients and nourishment. **Nutrients** are everything that you consume that can be used as energy. **Nourishment,** on the other hand, is the **energy** you get from nutrients plus the extra **information** that is in the food. Therefore, nourishment has quality included in it. When you eat a home-cooked meal, it is infinitely more nourishing for your body because it has **love** in it. A carefully prepared meal contains the chef's feelings for the person who will be eating it. If you eat at a restaurant or fast food place, the food does not have this aspect of information included in it.

Nourishment refers to how food affects you on **mental** and **spiritual** levels. If you see a great movie or watch your football team win a game, it is nourishing for your soul. Similarly, food can be good for your soul. To find out if food is nourishing, you need to ask yourself these questions: Where did the food come from? How was it grown? Who transported it? Who picked it?

Who cooked it? How was it cooked? If you can answer these questions, your food is healthier. You need more nourishing foods in your life. In fact, you need more nourishment in every part of your life if you want to improve your metabolism.

REDUCE YOUR TOXIC INPUT

One of the best ways to increase your metabolism is to reduce your intake of **toxins**. When toxins enter your body, you retain **water and fat** to dilute the ill effects that will result. This slows down your metabolism and makes you fat. The following inputs all contain harmful toxins. Try to eliminate them from your life to get healthy and boost your metabolic rate.

TAP WATER has chlorine and fluoride, both of which are extremely harmful to your body. Even taking a shower without filtering these minerals is toxic to your body. Drinking it is much worse.

ARTIFICIAL SWEETENERS such as aspartame (NutraSweet®), sucralose (Splenda®), high fructose corn syrup, and bleached white sugars and flours are extremely toxic. **Food taste enhancers** such as MSG (Monosodium Glutamate) are toxic as well.

TRANSFATS and hydrogenated oils are toxic and cancer causing. **Homogenized** and **pasteurized** milk cause heart disease. When meat products are irradiated with **radiation** beams to kill bacteria, they become very toxic too.

Many of the processed products from **fast food restaurants** are toxic. At home, when you over cook your food by microwaving or frying, you make the food toxic as well.

Some of most devastating **toxins** are the **non-prescription and prescription drugs** that you are taking. Unless and until you get off of these medications, you will not be able to improve your metabolism or your health. Your goal should be to slowly get off of all the medications you are taking. When you practice all the things that you have learned in this book, I am absolutely certain that you will be able to do it!

In your own body, you produce internal toxins like estrogen, which in high dosages can cause cancer. **Elemental toxins,** such as mercury in vaccines, aluminum in underarm deodorant, lead, arsenic, and silver, are also harmful in high doses. Synthetic toxins from chemical pesticides, petrochemical solvents, PBC, and dioxin are highly toxic as well.

You also need to make sure that you are not allergic to some of the most common allergy-causing foods. These foods are **milk and dairy products, wheat and grain products, corn, soy, peanuts, eggs,** and **strawberries.** When people with severe allergies and asthma conditions begin to stay away from these products, most of the time their conditions improve dramatically.

INCREASE ORGANIC RAW NUTRITION

More than 50 percent of the calories consumed by Americans are from processed foods like pasta, bread, bagels, sodas, and oils. Also, 40 percent of the average American diet is composed of animal products, which lack phytochemicals, flavinoids, antioxidants, and natural cofactors.[436] This kind of diet is dangerous and toxic for your health. Eating processed foods and animal products in excess is why you are **overeating**—you are not getting enough nutrients.

Many of my patients could not lose weight with other diet programs because they never received proper nutrients. They reduced their calories but were never satisfied and didn't lose weight. That's because when you deprive your body of proper nutrients, you will overeat to compensate. Your body is amazingly intelligent and knows it needs more nutrients. If you eat all organic foods, you will get the nutrients you need, so you will not overeat and you will increase your metabolism.

Organic foods have not been altered and processed by man, so they contain complete nutrients. Plants that are organic are raised without chemical fertilizers and herbicides; they are not genetically modified to produce more crops. **Organic animal products** are not raised with growth hormones or antibiotics, and they're not fed ground-up dead animals. They are allowed to roam free and eat natural grasses. These animals produce **free-ranged** meat.

EXERCISE AND MOVE

When the earth moves and the wind blows, your metabolism kicks into high gear. You must exercise to jumpstart your metabolism and lose weight. The reality is that you can eat all the best organic foods, but if you don't move and exercise, they will all sit in your stomach without being properly digested. Exercising is like cleaning your backyard with a motorized water jet cleaner. Once you power wash the filth away, your backyard will never look the same. Similarly, exercise will help your metabolism move fast, which will clean everything out of your body.

REDUCE STRESS

When you reduce your stress levels, you will increase your metabolism, guaranteed. A big part of stress comes of **sleep deprivation**. Sleeping seven to eight hours each night is crucial for speeding up your metabolism. Also, decreasing the **negative images** you see on the news, TV, video games, movies and in newspapers will help lower your stress levels. Listening to good music and using aromatherapy are also good for fighting stress. In addition, one of the best ways to beat stress and help your metabolism is to get a pet. Studies show that loving and petting an animal can drastically increase feelings of calm.

As I hope you've noticed throughout this book, the **spiritual aspects** of health are most important. Laughing regularly and often is lifesaving because it helps free your spirit. Giving and receiving many hugs, being thankful, being kind to strangers and loved ones, finding your purpose, and setting goals for yourself are all amazing ways to fight the ill effects of stress and improve your metabolism.

READ FOOD LABELS

Unfortunately, no one has had any training in reading food labels. We just don't learn how! But it's something we all need to do. I highly recommend taking the time to learn all the details about labeling practices for food products. Below, I have included a short overview of what you need to watch out for on labels, but I could spend a whole book talking about this subject. If you want to learn more, there are plenty of resources available on the Internet that will give you excellent information about labeling.

As we discussed earlier in this chapter, many of the artificial products in processed foods are extremely toxic to your body. There are so many that can hurt you, but the following toxic substances are particularly bad.

MSG (monosodium glutamate) is an extremely toxic food taste enhancer. It is an excitotoxin that makes our cells overexcited and causes them to fire uncontrollably. Eventually, this causes the death of the cells. MSG can cause autism, schizophrenia, seizures, brain tumors, Alzheimer's disease, cerebral palsy, episodic violence, and criminal behaviors.[437] MSG will also increase your appetite and make you gain weight. MSG and related toxins are added to foods disguised as "hydrolyzed vegetable protein," "vegetable protein," "natural flavorings," and "spices."[438] If you see these phrases on packaging, look out!

ASPARTAME is in almost all diet sodas. It is highly addicting. It is 200 times sweeter than sugar. It is in breakfast cereals, chewing gum, diet sodas, and is added to anything that says "sugar free" or "without sugar added."[439] Aspartame contains methanol, which is a wood alcohol that has toxic effects on the brain, optic nerves, and retinas.[440] It breaks down into phenylalanine and aspartic acid, both of which cause severe headaches, seizures, impairment of vision, dizziness, rashes, extreme fatigue, depression, a change of personality, confusion, memory loss, weight gain, diabetes, and many other diseases.[441]

HIGH FRUCTOSE CORN SYRUP is made of highly processed corn products. It is put in most packaged foods and regular sodas. High fructose corn syrup is highly addicting and fattening. It is in beverages, ice cream, candy, jam, ketchup, and baked goods.[442] It causes blood sugar problems, depression, fatigue, B vitamin deficiency, hyperactivity, indigestion, tooth decay, periodontal disease, and elevated triglycerides.[443]

TRANSFATS OR PARTIALLY HYDROGENATED OILS are the processed fats that last forever. They never go bad because they were never alive. Transfats cause heart disease and cancer—stay away from them! The presence of transfats is indicated by the phrase "partially hydrogenated" on food labels. Even if a product claims to have no transfats, it does if it contains these words. Transfats are in baked goods, cakes, cookies, instant soups, sauces, beef stew, corn chips, salad dressing, doughnuts, easy-to-spread butter, and margarine.[444] Hydrogenation deodorizes and bleaches the vegetable oil and chemically configures it to fool your cells. Transfats are pretenders, hardening cell walls and impeding flexibility and mobility of your cells.[445] Transfats are associated with heart disease, breast and colon cancer, atherosclerosis, elevated cholesterol, and numerous other diseases.[446]

WHITE SUGAR is processed sugar that is highly toxic and fattening. Like many of the substances on this list, it is also highly addictive.

NATURAL AND ARTIFICIAL FLAVORS are made of hundreds, if not thousands, of chemicals that don't have to be disclosed in the labels. When a label says a product contains natural flavors, don't believe there is anything natural about it. Obviously, when it says it is artificial, it is not good for you. Natural and artificial flavors may even contain toxic MSG.[447] They can also cause reproductive problems and developmental disorders.[448]

SPICES can be composed of hundreds of manmade, processed chemicals. "Spices" is a generic term used to protect trade secrets; the product may actually contain a combination of many different spices, or it may be fumigated or irradiated.[449]

ARTIFICIAL COLORS are in all the processed packaged goods. Any kind of dye on a label means the food is absolutely toxic to your body. "Red 7," "blue 14," and other color phrases signal dyes have been added. They cause hyperactivity in children, learning and visual disorders, nerve damage and cancer.[450]

ARTIFICIAL SWEETENERS are sucrose, saccharin, sucralose, dextrose, and many more.

SUCROSE (table sugar) is a disaccharide of glucose and fructose. It is chemically processed and bleached. Sucrose is highly toxic and addictive. It causes blood sugar problems, depression, fatigue, B vitamin deficiency, hyperactivity, tooth decay, periodontal disease, and indigestion.[451]

SACCHARIN (Sweet 'N Low®) is in beverages, candy, table sweeteners, chewing gum, jams, jellies, chewable aspirin, toothpaste, and pharmaceutical preparations. It causes diarrhea, eczema, nausea, hives, headache, cancer, and developmental and reproductive disorders.[452]

SUCRALOSE (Splenda®) is chlorinated sugar. It caused thymus gland shrinkage, enlarged liver and kidneys, and diarrhea in animal studies. It contains dangerous contaminants, such as heavy metals, methanol, arsenic, and others.[453]

DEXTROSE is in corn syrup. Please see the above section on high fructose corn syrup.

FOOD IRRADIATION is bombarding food with ionizing radiation to kill bacteria. It destroys vitamins and minerals and kills all living cells in the irradiated food. If you see the label below, you need to avoid the product. During the irradiation process, chemical reactions cause the formation of harmful chemicals like formaldehyde and benzene, both of which can lead to cancer.[454]

SIX METHODS FOR DETOXIFICATION

Detoxification happens when bad things come out of your body. You can let go of toxins through the following six methods of elimination, which you can see in the illustration on page 235. Every time you get toxins out of your body in one of these ways, you help increase your metabolism.

1. URINATION. Your body eliminates water and other fluids through urination. All urine contains toxins, which were filtered out of your blood by your kidneys and liver. When you super hydrate, you will be able to eliminate all the toxins in your body's fluids because you will urinate more often.

2. BOWEL MOVEMENTS. Protein, sugar, fat, and fiber are removed from your body through bowel movements. Your liver, stomach, and intestines are responsible for filtering the toxins that are eventually eliminated in this way. I recommend periodic cleansings to make sure you get everything out. You can get all kinds of cleansings, including lymphatic, parasitic, candida, colon, liver, gallbladder, heavy metal, and kidney and bladder cleansings, all of which will eliminate toxins. I also recommend fasting periodically or taking salt baths.

3. SWEATING. Minerals and other smaller particles are eliminated through this route. Since your skin is the largest organ of your body, sweating is the most effective way to detoxify because of the sheer volume of sweat produced. When you exercise and sweat regularly, you will be able to use this way of detoxification to its fullest potential. Spending time in an infrared sauna is another way to eliminate some toxins through sweating.

4. BREATHING, VOMITING, COUGHING, SNEEZING, AND RUNNY NOSE. Toxins from your lungs are excreted through your mouth and nose in the methods listed above. That is why exercise is important; it eliminates these toxins through deep breathing. When you have too many toxins in your lungs, your body gets sick to get rid of them. In other words, **your illness is the cure** for your toxicity. Sometimes, the contents of your stomach can come out through vomiting, which is quite an emergency! It shows that your body doesn't want the toxic foods you eat.

5. CRYING. Tears are sometimes the most effective way to express emotions. Whether you are happy, sad, or terrified, tears are released to eliminate your emotional toxins. I encourage you to have more crying sessions; let yourself get emotional with touching movies, good conversations, faith based services, or other activities.

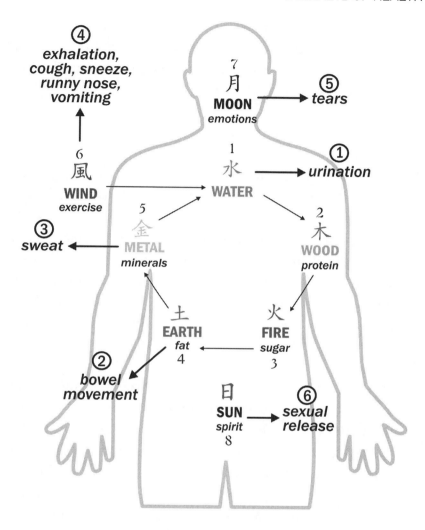

6 Ways of Elimination/Detoxification

6. SEXUAL RELEASE. Contrary to how most people view it, sexual intimacy is a spiritual act of creating love. This is why it is called "lovemaking." Of course, there is physical pleasure and emotional sharing associated with sex. But above all, it is the ultimate expression of love and our life-giving ability. Sexual release is what's required to create a new life. This intimacy of

235

lovemaking bears no judgment, no shame, and is done with complete trust. This is the kind of intimacy that I talked about in the emotional trauma section; when you don't have this kind of intimacy, you will be traumatized.

9 CAUSES OF DISEASES

In my research, I have realized that there are only nine things that cause every disease known to mankind. There are many symptoms—thousands of ailments with different names—but only nine reasons for these problems. And I believe there is only one cure for all these diseases. It is beyond the scope of this book to elaborate in depth, but I will go into more detail in my upcoming book called *9 Secrets of Disease—9 Causes, Many Symptoms and 1 Cure*. For now, I have listed the nine causes briefly below.

CAUSE #1: OXIDATION. Oxidation is the process behind **aging**. When a banana ages, it turns from green to yellow, yellow to brown, and brown to black; all of these changes are caused by the acidifying effects of oxidation. Oxidation is literally rust in some cases; when metal objects rust, they have been oxidized.

The effects of oxygen in your body aren't as noticeable, but they still happen. When oxygen goes into your body and burns your food as fuel, it produces free radicals.[455] Free radicals are the atoms that lose their electrons when they interact with oxygen. They are looking to recapture the electrons to be stabilized, so they attack other molecules to take them. They come when you overeat, are stressed, lack sleep, lack exercise, and even when you are just plain breathing and living. You can counteract oxidation and free radical damage with antioxidants like **vitamins A, C, E, D** and **glutathione**.[456]

Antioxidants have extra electrons to donate to free radicals, which calms effects of oxidation and aging.

CAUSE #2: MALNUTRITION. Most Americans are malnourished. They are eating lots of food, but it's all the wrong things. As discussed before, processed foods have no nutrients or live enzymes. They are filled with toxins like refined sugar, high fructose corn syrup, transfats, processed milk and cheese, and many other artificial products. They lack phytonutrients, fiber, vitamins, minerals and co-factors.[457] In order to cure this problem, you need to eat more **organic raw foods**. You also need to stay away from manmade products as much as you can. You need to rebuild yourself with good materials, not trash!

CAUSE #3: INFLAMMATION. All the artificial sweeteners, food enhancers, and preservatives you eat can cause severe allergic reactions in your body. Ultimately, these things can lead to diseases such as cancer, hypertension, diabetes, and more. Food allergens, heavy metals, microbes, lack of exercise and lack of sleep will cause inflammation of your cells.[458] You need to cleanse your digestive system with colon, liver, gallbladder, candida, parasite, and kidney cleanses. You also need to help digestion by supplementing probiotics, fiber, hydrochloric acid, and enzymes. Practice eating green, green, greens to cool down the effect of this fire.

CAUSE #4: IMPAIRED METABOLISM. This is a result of everything you learned in this chapter. **Poor eating habits**, lack of exercise, and insufficient rest are the main culprits behind impaired metabolisms.[459] When your metabolism doesn't function properly, your wheel of life is just not turning. You need to improve your eating, exercising, thinking, and feeling habits to overcome this problem.

CAUSE #5: IMPAIRED DETOXIFICATION. We talked about detoxification at the beginning of this chapter. Lack of detoxification is devastating for your metabolism and health. When you overload on food allergens, non-prescription and prescription medications, heavy metals, environmental, internal, and chemical toxins, your metabolism will become sluggish. First, you will get fat, and then you'll get sick. You need to remove all the allergens and toxins from your diet and repair your digestive and urinary tracks to fix this problem.

CAUSE #6: STRUCTURAL TRAUMA. This problem happens when the structure of your body is out of alignment. Structural trauma starts in two different places, as we discussed in the exercise chapter. When your feet are out of alignment from lack of walking, the rest of your body is affected and gets out of position too. Similarly, when you **sit too long**, your hip joints get out of alignment, causing all kinds of back and other structural problems. You need to strengthen your muscles, walk more, and sit less to fight this very insidious cumulative trauma.

CAUSE #7: PHYSICAL TRAUMA. When you have accidents that result in bleeding skin, broken bones, and other serious problems, you will obviously be at greater risk for bigger physical ailments. In these cases, you need emergency care consisting of medications and even surgery. You will also need to rehabilitate to get back to your regular routine.

CAUSE #8: EMOTIONAL TRAUMA. As you learned in the emotional trauma section of this book, emotional wounds are very undertreated medical problems. I truly believe that emotional trauma is what shapes your behaviors. You need to heal from your old wounds and your current wounds that are wreaking havoc on your body, mind, and spirit. You need to freely share your old trauma that is ruining your life to transform into a new you. You need to overcome this emotional trauma to get healthy. You need to participate in seminars or sessions where you can truly learn to share and release your wounds as soon as you can.

CAUSE #9: SPIRITUAL TRAUMA. This kind of trauma occurs when you are disconnected from your creator. Your parents are not your creators. They are the factory workers who just participated in assembling you. They had no idea what they were doing when they made you. If they knew, they would not have made you the way you are.

You are mistaken to think that you are made from some type of random accident. You are designed to have an **intimate relationship with your creator**, God. Not having this relationship is why most people cannot attain the perfect health that they were designed to have. If you think not having parents or not being loved was a bad enough kind of trauma, then you don't realize how important a relationship with God is in your life. You are in big trouble when you don't accept love from your creator. This is the most urgent medical condition, one which you need to attend to immediately.

SCHEDULE YOUR HEALTH

Look at the ideal timeline of how you should perform daily tasks to boost your metabolism. Now, draw in the methods you use throughout your day in the blank clock on the right.

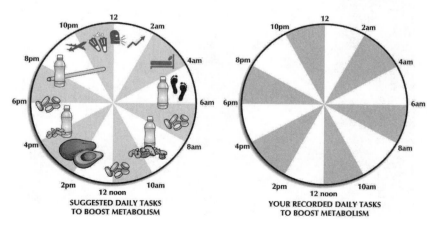

SUGGESTED DAILY TASKS
TO BOOST METABOLISM

YOUR RECORDED DAILY TASKS
TO BOOST METABOLISM

METABOLISM WELLNESS SCORING CHART

How do you measure up? Circle what you do to boost your metabolism on the following chart. Give yourself one point if more of your circles fall above the dotted line. If you have multiple circles below the line, you need to reevaluate your eating habits.

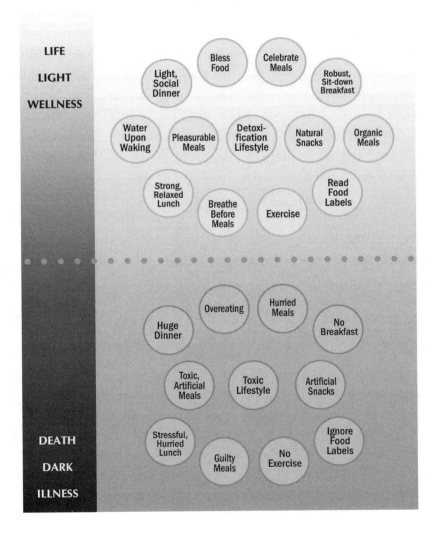

Metabolism Wellness Scoring Chart
Circle what you do to boost your metabolism

Chapter 11

THE MASTER SECRET:
HEART

"JUST BELIEVE"

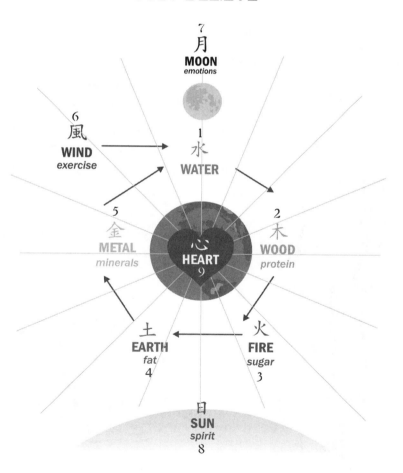

Only with heart can man believe in righteousness. This is known as faith. Having heart is the master element in the system of the universe. If you don't accept the changes that I've talked about with your heart, then nothing will happen to you. But if you commit your heart to a healthy life, you'll see miracles happen. You know in your head that God gave you all the power to heal yourself from any disease. If you accept this in your heart, you will transform your life into one of wellness. So just believe!

IMPORTANT HEART

Most people think the brain has control over the body, but, really, the heart influences everything we do. You need your heart to stay alive. The pumping of your heart is how your body gets the oxygen it needs. Your heart beats about 100,000 times each day! That's approximately 40 million beats each year and 3 billion beats over the average lifetime. Your heart is also the first organ to develop; it starts

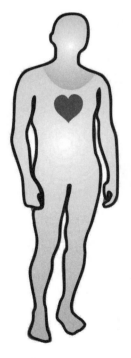

Your Heart's Response

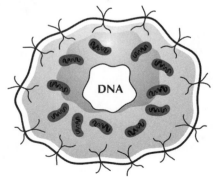

Your Cell's Response

beating just a few weeks after conception![460] Your brain is the second organ to develop in your body.

The heart also has an amazing ability that the brain doesn't share—entrainment. **Entrainment** means that the heart can set everything in the same order. The concept was first discovered by clockmaker Christiaan Huygens in the 17th century. Huygens invented the pendulum clock and accumulated quite a collection in his studio. One night, he noticed that all the pendulums were swinging at the same time! Huygens tried misaligning the clock pendulums, but after a while, they began swinging in time once again. The clockmaker couldn't explain this strange phenomenon. Later researchers figured out that the largest pendulum clock electromagnetically had the power to lull the others into alignment with it. They termed this concept entrainment.[461]

Many living and nonliving things are affected by the principle of entrainment. Flocks of birds flying together and schools of fish swimming in the same direction are good examples of the concept at work. Women's menstrual cycles can also become entrained when many females live in close quarters.[462] Because of entrainment, your heart has the power to control all the functions in your body, even your brain. Through entrainment, your heart can set the brain in a rhythm, but the brain can't do the same for the heart. Your heart has an electromagnetic field that is **5,000 times** stronger than that of the brain; it reaches eight to 10 feet from your body![463] Because of this, your heart can entrain things outside your body too. It can reach out and touch other people's hearts.

INDEPENDENT HEART

Another reason your heart is the most important part of your body is that it's independent from your brain. If you were to receive a **heart transplant,** there would be no way for doctors to reconnect the vagus nerve, which connects the heart to the brain.[464] The heart would function on its own, without guidance from the brain.[465] This happens in people who haven't had a heart transplant too. Many studies performed by Dr. J. Armour in 1991 proved that when the brain sends messages to the heart, the heart does not always obey. Contrarily, when the heart sends signals to the brain, the brain always responds.[466]

Dr. Armour discovered there's actually a **brain in the heart** itself. Your heart has about 40,000 neurons of its own, which allow it to work independently of your brain. It's the heart that decides, not the brain. The heart supersedes the brain.

YOUR HEART'S RESPONSE

Hearts are very interactive organs. They take things personally. Your heart can respond positively or negatively in your body and cells, as you can see in the following illustration.

Look over the chart on the next page to compare your heart's response to the elements of the moon and sun. [467]

As you can see, if you are filled with **negative emotions,** like those represented by the moon, your heart will be put under stress. Feelings of hatred, anger, resentment, revenge, fear, blame, and selfishness cause a physical response in your body, including in your heart; your blood vessels shrink, levels of stress hormones increase, your immune system becomes less effective, and your heart rate increases. In a stressful environment, your heart also stops beating regularly. It works inconsistently, which makes your whole body less efficient.

Your heart responds to **positive information** as well. When your life is filled with the light of the sun—wisdom, love,

YOUR HEART'S RESPONSE	
MOON (Emotional)	**SUN (Spiritual)**
Knowledge, hatred, anger, resentment, revenge, fear, blame, selfishness	Wisdom, love, appreciation, joy, non-judgment, patience, forgiveness, tolerance
Blood vessels shrink, 30 negative stress hormones are released, 1400 negative reactions take place, immune system effectiveness reduced	Blood vessels open, stress hormones diminish, immune system more effective
Heart rate goes up, heart beats inconsistently	Heart rate slows, heart beats consistently, heart entrains other organs to be steady as well
HRV — **ANGER** (Heart Rate)	HRV — **APPRECIATION** (Heart Rate)

appreciation, joy, non judgment, patience, forgiveness and tolerance—your heart opens up. It works better with positive information, beating more consistently and at a slower rate. And when your heart beats regularly, it trains the rest of your organs to function well too. Just by looking at your heart's beat pattern, you can tell that anger isn't good for it. **Heart rate variability (HRV)** is a measurement of beat-to-beat changes in the heart rate. HRV rhythms have consistently emerged as the most dynamic heart monitors. They're reflective of your inner emotional status.[468] Notice the two patterns in the chart. Which one seems healthier?

When you listen and follow your heart, your thoughts will become more intelligent, your decisions will be more educated, and your emotions will be more balanced and coherent.[469] Your heart will also stay physically in shape. Help your heart beat regularly, and it will stay healthy longer.

EXERCISE YOUR HEART

If you make an effort to bring loving feelings into your heart, your entire body will respond. Try the following heart lock-in exercise as a way to use your heart's entrainment abilities to your advantage:[470]

Do this exercise whenever you feel stressed out to achieve a feeling of calm and inner peace.

EXERCISE: HEART LOCK-IN

1. Find a quiet place. Close your eyes and relax.

2. Focus your energy toward your heart. Don't think about your head or other parts of your body. Pretend to breathe through your heart.

3. Concentrate on someone easy to love and appreciate for five to 15 minutes. Remember how this person made you feel. Keep breathing love and care through your heart.

4. Gently send out the sense of love and appreciation that you are experiencing to other people.

5. Feel softness in your heart. Focus back to your heart and repeat the first part of this exercise if you feel blocked energy.

6. Write down any intuitive thoughts you gained for future use:

_____

_____

_____

FINDING MEANING IN YOUR LIFE

Your genes respond to meaning and need. If you don't give meaning to your existence, your own immune system, specifically your T cells, will attack your cells and destroy them. This can happen in many different areas of your body. Your body is so efficient that it will destroy what you don't need.

The medical term for self destruction in the cells is **autoimmune disease.** There are over 80 diseases caused by autoimmunity.

Some of the well known ones are rheumatoid arthritis, lupus, multiple sclerosis, psoriasis, type I diabetes, Crohn's disease and ankylosing spondylitis. These are chronic, life-threatening issues. Unfortunately, the only medical solution for these diseases right now is debilitating immunosuppressive medications. However, when you find your purpose and give yourself a reason for existence, many of these diseases will improve dramatically without medical treatment.

Dr. Viktor Frankl is the iconic example of someone with a purpose. He lived through the Holocaust in a Nazi concentration camp. He wanted to publish his manuscript, so he forced himself to keep living. Most of the other prisoners in the camp were depressed and couldn't handle the pain, so they committed suicide by not eating. Only 10 percent of the people came out alive. Most didn't have any reason to live. After Dr. Frankl was freed from the prison camp, he thought about his will to live. He eventually published a book about it, inventing a new form of psychological therapy called logotherapy. "Logos" means purpose or meaning in Greek, and Dr. Frankl's new philosophy dealt with the power of purpose in life. **Logotherapy** teaches that even the tragic and negative aspects of life, such as unavoidable suffering, can be turned into a human achievement with the right attitude.[471] In other words, when you find your meaning, you will heal from your ailments.

Dr. Frankl's solution to almost all problems is simple: we must will a meaning to our lives. As Friedrich Nietzche once said, "He who has a 'why' to live for can bear almost any 'how.'" Once we find a meaning—a reason to be happy and successful—happiness and success will ensue. It's a cycle, and we have to *pursue* meaning before results will *ensue*. In other words, if you want to be happy, don't try to find happiness. You should first have a reason to be happy; after that, happiness will follow naturally.[472]

FINDING PURPOSE IN YOUR LIFE

Your heart is home to your overriding purpose for life; it motivates you to keep going and try to achieve your goals. But not every heart has a purpose. It's a shame, but many people I talk to claim they don't have a reason for living. I felt that way too before I found my true **purpose through God**. God is really the key to success in life and the master key to health—accept God into your life, find your purpose in your heart, and health will follow. All that you've learned in this book will be useless if you don't have a purpose.

If you were told to find a landmark in a city you had never visited, would you be able to get there? You might stumble upon the destination after searching for a long time, but you probably wouldn't find it on your first try. Unless you have detailed directions and a plan in mind, it's hard to reach an unfamiliar destination. The same holds true for your life purpose. If you don't know where you're going or how to get there, you'll just wander aimlessly through life. You might eventually find yourself in a good place, but you probably won't get there at first.

To avoid a directionless coast through life, we need to have a purpose. And in order to achieve your purpose, you have to constantly reevaluate your situation. If you're driving to a landmark, you have to change your movements based on your current location. Similarly, you always need to adjust your actions in life to reach your goals depending on where you stand. Ask yourself all the time, "Where am I going? Why am I going there?" In his book, *The Seven Habits of Highly Effective People*, Dr. Stephan Covey says to "begin with the end in mind." Take his advice and have a clear plan laid out for your life. Know where you want to end up—have a purpose—and assess your progress regularly.

THE FOUR QUALITIES OF PURPOSE

Your purpose in life can't be a vague idea of what you want. No, you need to have a blueprint laid out and ready. You wouldn't start building a house without a blueprint; why build your life without one? There are four qualities that every purpose should have; it should be **obtainable, challenging, measurable,** and **strategic. Obtainable** just means that your purpose shouldn't be out of reach; in other words, don't make your goal something that you know is impossible. At the same time, however, your purpose should **challenge** you—it needs to stretch your limits. Hard work is required to reach any good purpose. **Measurable** means that you can track your progress; you want to have multiple, small goals to reach so you don't get discouraged. Finally, your reason for living needs to be **strategic.** That means you should have a plan as to exactly how you will achieve your goals. A good method for forming a purpose is to complete this sentence: I'm going to be _____, and I plan to get there by _____.

People who have a clear blueprint that's obtainable, challenging, measurable, and strategic are much more likely to be successful in their lives. A study of the Yale University class of 1960 proved this point. At the time of their graduation, a poll showed that only three percent of the Yale graduates had detailed, written plans for the future. Twenty years later, when the same class was resurveyed, this same three percent had more assets than the remaining 97 percent combined. Obviously, it pays to have a clear purpose.

PURPOSE FINDER QUESTIONS

Use the following questions to find your life's purpose. Think about each category carefully, and then use the qualities from each section to develop a statement of meaning for your life. You will probably be stumped at first; that's okay. Try to do the exercise over and over again until you can develop a statement. I guarantee that it will become easier each time you do it. Once you've found a purpose, bring it into your heart. Use the heart lock-in exercise I mentioned earlier in this chapter to set your heart on your goals. Memorize and mesmerize your purpose; say it to yourself every day. If you put your heart into it, everything you need will come true.

Your statement should sum up want you want to make of yourself. For an example, I'll share my purpose with you: I'm here to educate, empower, and inspire everyone to get back on their feet in the areas of health, success, business, finance, career, and relationships. I repeat this purpose like a mantra every day. You should do that too—keep saying your statement and you'll attract it. You'll magnetize your life so that you get what you want.

The most influential book in my life has been *The Purpose Driven Life* by Pastor Rick Warren. I have read this book nine

---

EXERCISE: PURPOSE FINDER QUESTIONS

Passion: What do I love to do?

Talent: What am I good at?

Personality: What am I like?

Experience: What have I been through?

Spiritual Gifts: What has been given to me?

Use your answers to form a one sentence purpose statement for your life:

---

times so far, and I plan to read it at least once every year from now on. The most profound thing it has taught me is in the very first chapter. Here, Pastor Warren tells us a simple truth: **"It all starts from God."**[473] This is where most of us fail. We all start from us. But we don't have the answers to our problems. Without God, we are lost. He designed us and created us for His purpose. He is where all power comes from.

PASSIONATE HEART

If you find your true meaning and purpose in life, you will become **passionate** about all that you do. You will be like a magnet, attracting the love and admiration of everyone around you. You will be that person who everyone wants to be around. You will become unstoppable in your mission to accomplish your purpose. But in order to have all this, you need to love what you do and follow your true purpose.

Unfortunately, most of the people I know do not love what they do. They work because they have to, but they don't enjoy their jobs. This is a tragedy! You need to find what you love to do and discover a way to make this your work. Then, you will be passionate. One way to find out if you are truly passionate about your job is to ask yourself a single question: **"Would I still do what I do even if I didn't get paid to do it?"** If you wouldn't work your job without pay, you haven't yet found your ideal work. I hope and pray that eventually, you find your passion.

MANAGING YOUR HEART ENERGY

Think of your heart's energy as a bank account. When your heart account is balanced and well maintained, you save energy and benefit. When your heart is out of balance, you lose energy and suffer. When you learn to manage and monitor the energy bank account in your heart, you can be truly healthy.[474] Continuing the bank metaphor, think of **energy assets** as the events that are energizing and harmonious. **Energy deficits,** on the other hand, are those events that feel incoherent, disharmonious, and draining.[475]

The best way to manage your heart energy is to find what makes you happy—what gives you positive energy—and to do more of those things. Read over this list of energy gainers and

MY ENERGY GAINERS	MY ENERGY DRAINERS
__ Speaking my truth	__ Sugar
__ Quality time with kids	__ Caffeine
__ Being honest	__ Not exercising
__ Following through with commitments	__ Arguing with my spouse or loved ones
__ Reading good books	__ Stress
__ Keeping promises to myself	__ Drama
__ Being grateful for my blessings	__ Interruptions
__ Prayer	__ Being overweight
__ Eating healthy	__ Overworking
__ Taking my supplements everyday	__ Over scheduling my day
__ Date night with my spouse	__ Saying yes when I mean no
__ Quality time with friends	__ Not taking play time
__ Focusing on the positive	__ Taking abuse
__ Having faith	__ Worrying too much
__ Expressing gratitude	__ Slouching
__ Standing up for myself	__ Overanalyzing
__ Staying on task	__ Trying to change other people
__ Letting go of things out of my control	__ Being a people pleaser
__ Taking action when it comes to my goals	__ Stressing out
__ Making time to exercise	__ Watching mindless television
__ Getting regular foot care	__ Not having a purpose
__ Maintaining good posture	__ Not completing things that I start
__ Massages	__ Mindless internet surfing
__ Saving money	__ Eating pre-packaged or prepared meals
__ Being involved with causes I believe in	
__ Celebrating special occasions	

drainers, and choose the qualities that apply to you. Use the list as a starting point, adding your own energy descriptions as they come to mind. After you identify your pleasures and pains, I'll discuss ways to manage your energy so you experience more positive gainers than negative drainers.[476]

Which do you have more of, drainers or gainers? If you have more things that drain your positive energy, think about why this is so. Is there any way you could reduce these draining activities? Make a commitment to change your behaviors for the better! After you've examined your drainers, take a look at your list of energy gainers. Focus on each of these activities for a moment. What about each one makes you happy? Next, think about whether you could increase your participation in any of these things. Finally, look over the items on the list that you did not check. Are any of these other gainers appealing to you? If so, try incorporating them into your routine. You can never do too many things that make you happy.

PLACEBOS, THE SUGAR PILLS

In Latin, placebo means "I will please." The term was first used to describe priests who sang for the dead. Usually, the priests were not nearly as affected by death as the loved ones of the person who died. Still, the priests tried to console the sufferers by sharing in the mourning.[477] They didn't have any substance to their sadness, but because they seemed to be mourning, they made the real sufferers feel much better. The same concept holds true for placebos in the drug world. Sugar pills don't have any substance to them—they're just sugar—but when people *think* they're real, they can give the same results as an actual drug.

Physicians know about the power of placebos and have used them to treat patients for centuries. But recently, placebos have been used mostly as dummy medications and as controls for clinical trials that are designed to test "real" drugs.[478] Randomized, placebo-controlled, double-blind experiments are designed to answer one question—will an experimental treatment produce better results than the placebo? If the results from the treatment are better than the placebo, it is deemed effective.[479] Unfortunately, many of the drugs or treatments tested do not work better than placebos, but they're still available for consumers. Shockingly, more than half of the clinical trials for the six leading antidepressants did not outperform placebos.[480]

The fact that so many clinical trials fail to meet the placebo's level of effectiveness isn't surprising. Placebos are **extraordinary drugs.** They work in at least a third of patients and sometimes in as many as 60 percent of those who try them.[481] But placebos only work when patients believe they will work. They prove the **power of belief!** Unfortunately, modern medicine scoffs at the idea of using placebos as a drug; nowadays, the only place for sugar pills is in clinical trials. Since conventional medicine bases its approach on science, it tends to disregard faith-based treatments. In fact, conventional medicine tends to view faith and placebo effects as neither reliable nor provable.[482]

In reality, placebos can be more powerful than potent drugs. Sometimes, they can even reverse the actions of conventional treatments. In some studies, placebo-based reactions are almost 100 percent effective![483] And even when results are not purely from a placebo, its effects can be felt. The placebo effect is part of every treatment; factors such as the circumstances of the patients and the authority, character, and personality of the healing professional can make a big difference in treatment results, and all of these things have to do with belief.[484] In fact, the most important aspect of any placebo treatment is the relationship between the healer and the patient.[485]

PLACEBOS, THE BELIEF EFFECT

The placebo effect is an effect with no external cause; it is purely a **function of faith**.[486] Ultimately, it is the belief in the treatment that sets off the placebo response.[487] When you believe that something will work so much so that your belief is part of your consciousness, what you have is no longer a belief or an idea but faith. The placebo, then, is when an idea about your health becomes your faith.[488] When the placebo effect works, it means you have been cured by nothing but your own faith in the cure. It is a miracle that anyone can perform, a **self healing**.[489]

Faith is a deep knowing—an unwavering acceptance that something is true.[490] The placebo effect is a manifestation of faith. It allows you to see something of your own power and the power of believing. The source of this power is God.[491] When you receive God's power and believe in it in your heart, you will be able to truly heal your mind, body, and spirit.

NOCEBOS, THE BELIEF EFFECT

The placebo effect refers to the positive power of belief, but there can also be **negative belief**—the nocebo effect. When your mind is engaged in negative suggestions that can damage your health, the negative effects are collectively referred to as the nocebo effect.[492] Most often, the harmful nocebo effect is caused by a bad doctor/patient relationship.[493] And unfortunately, negative nocebo effects are just as powerful as positive placebo effects. For example, if your doctor tells you that you have only three months to live with your terminal cancer, it is very likely that you will not live much longer than that. In your mind, you will believe that three months are all you have, so you will, in a way, will yourself to death!

The nocebo effect works because, unfortunately, your authority figures like doctors, parents, and teachers make you believe that you are powerless.[494] This is a devastating result of modern medicine. The development of technology and science in medicine has led to less contact between doctors and patients. A caring doctor/patient relationship is hard to find nowadays. We must find ways to restore healing relationships between patients and healers for positive belief effects to take precedence over negative ones; that means that doctors and other health professionals will have to try to maintain positive attitudes and develop feelings of empathy when dealing with ill patients.[495]

GOD'S SARANG, GOD'S SARAM

"Heart," as I've talked about it thus far, refers to our organs and our commitment to a meaningful life. But it also means **faith**. All that I've presented in this book will change your life if you work hard for it. But the simple act of accepting God into your life will change your health more than anything—that's why heart is the **master key**. If you have faith, anything is possible. I know this from personal experience.

As I already told you in a previous chapter, my whole life was once driven by fear of failure and poverty. I have been going to church since I came to this country when I was 16 years old. Over a 30-year period, I went to church and watched spiritual people praising God and singing with their hands up in the air. I wondered what happened to them. Why didn't I feel the way they felt? For years, I didn't feel anything remarkable at church. That all changed when my father-in-law, who was a retired minister at All Nations Church, invited my wife and me to his church one Sunday in 2002. There, I heard Senior Pastor Yoo for the first time. I felt like I had been hit with a hammer. He sounded so different from any other pastor I had ever listened to. I decided to buy all of his tapes on every subject he taught. They were all amazing!

One day shortly afterward, I was listening to one of his programs while driving to work on the 710 freeway. Quite suddenly, I saw red blood pouring all over my body. When this blood touched my head, I felt an electrocuting sensation that swept over my whole body from head to toe. At this moment, I felt a message in my heart very clearly: "Son, have peace." As soon as I felt these words, I started to cry. Actually, I started balling. I don't know how I managed to get through rush-hour traffic and make it to work, but eventually, I found myself in my office parking lot. Although I was crying, I felt calmer and more at peace than ever before. I was so happy! I didn't want it to end. Unfortunately, I had patients waiting almost an hour for me because I spent that long in the car without realizing it. Reluctantly, I had to wipe away all my tears and get to work.

Later, I realized that I had received the **Holy Spirit** that morning in my car. I was listening to Pastor Yoo's Inner Healing seminar, in which he discusses emotional trauma and how the blood of Jesus can heal deep emotional wounds and fear. Apparently, this was the message that I needed to hear to heal my emotional wounds. I had done plenty of Bible studying during my years at Catholic high school and a Catholic college. I had abundant knowledge in God, but the real message of God didn't reach me until that morning. For the first time in my life, I actually wanted to read the Bible. Since then, I have been reading the Bible every day and, amazingly, I began to understand it for the first time. I was truly born again!

After my message, I felt God's Sarang (love) for the first time. I became God's Saram (person) for the first time too. It was not about me anymore; it was, and still is, all about God and what he wants me to do for the rest of my life. I no longer have to work so hard on my own. I no longer have to live in constant fear. He is with me and is guiding me every step of the way. He is my designer and creator. He is in complete control of my life. What a relief! All of my heavy burdens were completely lifted on that day. I felt such a relief that I cried out of joy and peace.

As soon as I received the Holy Spirit, I started dreaming of something new. This new dream was grander than I ever thought possible because I was no longer afraid. I didn't have any more limitations. It was simple: I wanted to be God's messenger of wellness. All the research and the studying I had been doing seemed to fall into place; my dream was to teach the whole world how to get well by receiving God's love and power. Since I had received His love and become a new person, I wanted to help others do the same. This had become my mission, purpose, and passion in life.

YOUR PERSONAL RELATIONSHIP WITH GOD.

You need to have a personal relationship with God. When it comes down to it, developing your relationship with your creator is your ultimate purpose in life. Having a relationship with God means feeling the heart of God in your own heart. This should be the basis for all the relationships of your life.

When you don't receive God's love on a consistent basis, you will suffer from the lack of love that we talked about in Chapter 8. In time, love sicknesses will create a void in your life. Keep your life fulfilled by holding intimate conversations with God, by listening to Him through meditation, by reading scriptures, by praying, worshiping, praising, and participating in other spiritual activities. Many people engage in religious activities and go to church, but they do not have personal relationship with God. Without a relationship with your creator, church activities are absolutely tiring and meaningless. I strongly urge you to develop an intimate relationship with God as soon as possible. It will change your life. Attend spiritual retreats offered by local churches to renew your spirit and be reborn.

JUST BELIEVE

Some 20 years ago, I read a book by Napoleon Hill titled *Think and Grow Rich*. This book changed my life at the time. It said that through the creative imagination of the mind, finite man has direct communication with infinite intelligence.[496] Back then, I realized for the first time that anything could be possible if I set my mind to it. That book became my Bible for the next 13 years until I received the Holy Spirit. After my revelation, I realized that it is **not willpower but faith** in God that makes one grow rich in every aspect of life. I now truly understand the real success that Napoleon Hill was talking about.

The problem with **willpower** is that it is too weak. It changes with time and situations. It takes too much energy and is exhausting. As I shared with you when I discussed my emotional fear, I lived with strong willpower all my life. But I was too stressed and too wired to achieve my own success. Willpower is flawed because it is self centered. It is all about you and nothing else. On the other hand, **faith** is strong and perpetual. It is selfless and God centered. This is why it is easy and constant. Once you depend on God for all your needs, you don't have to work that hard anymore. You will be empowered by His almighty being because you are plugged into Him. You become a conduit of His power to achieve His purpose through your life. All this happens when you decide to **just believe**.

Right now, you are **bound** by your own negative thoughts and emotions. Your thoughts are limited by manmade messages you received by your upbringing. Your wounded emotions of rejection, anger, fear, hunger, inferiority, and guilt in the past are constantly controlling your life. This is the true darkness of your life. No matter how healthy you eat and drink, no matter how well you exercise and move, this moment of darkness will destroy your health instantly. You need to bring in the love of God, the light, to chase away your darkness in every waking moment of your life. This is the ultimate truth that Jesus talked about in the Gospel of John 8:32 "Then you will know the truth, and the truth will set you free." When you receive the light of God, you will truly be **free** and heal from all your diseases of body, mind, and spirit.

Animals have instincts. Tiny salmon are born in streams, swim to the ocean, and then, in four years, make the arduous upstream journey to the exact spot where they were born. Elephants go back to where they came from when it's their time to die. These animals are programmed and have no choice in their fate. But we have conscious minds that can choose. Our free will is evidence of the true love of God. He loves us so much that He gives us freedom to choose our paths. He respects us so much that he gives us choices. He could have programmed us like other animals, but instead, He gave us power to make our own destiny. WOW!

"Don't be afraid. Just believe." This is a common verse in the Bible. In fact, scripture tells us not to be afraid 366 times in its pages. The Bible teaches us not to fear enough for each day in the year and one more time just to make sure we get it right. And the Bible gives us the cure for fear right after it tells us to stop being afraid; that cure is to **just believe.** When you just believe, you will not be afraid anymore. So choose to just believe. I believe that since we are made in the image of God, we are creators of our own universe, just like He is. The Creator God made the infinite universe, and we, His creatures, can choose to create a certain universe of our own.

Which universe will you choose? Will you choose life or death? Will you choose light or darkness? Will you choose wellness or illness? Will you choose your heart or your head? Will you choose a union with God or a union with the material world? Will you choose the eternal spirit or the temporal body? Will you choose happiness or unhappiness? Will you choose love or fear?

God created our universe, and it is your turn to create your own universe the way you want to . . . it is all up to you. When you learn of God's unconditional love in your head and believe it in your heart, then **hope** comes. This hope is called the belief factor, and it can truly spark God's energy to transform your life into one of wellness. It will happen in every level of your universe, at the quantum, atomic, cellular, bodily, solar, and galactic levels. To "just believe" means that God gave you all the power to heal yourself from any disease. When you receive this power of belief, you will be able to heal everything from the common cold to cancer and any disease in between.

I would like to testify to you how I transformed my life through God's love at my seminars. Will you join me?

SCHEDULE YOUR HEART HEALTH

Look at the charts on the following page. The one on the left lists all the activities you should do to take care of your heart. How do you compare to this ideal? Draw in your heart-healthy activities on the blank chart to the right.

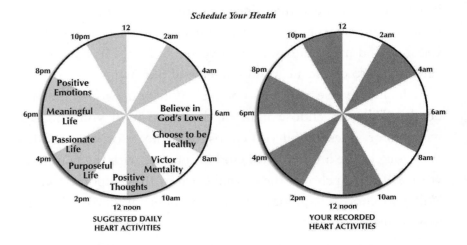

Schedule Your Health

SUGGESTED DAILY
HEART ACTIVITIES

YOUR RECORDED
HEART ACTIVITIES

HEART WELLNESS SCORING CHART

Circle what your heart decides to do on the following chart. Give yourself one point if more of your circles are above the dotted line.

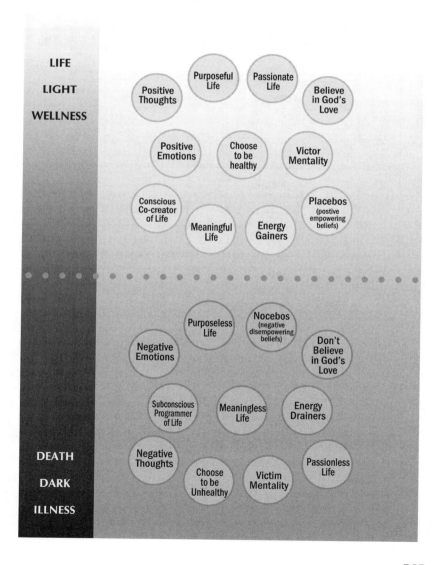

Heart Wellness Scoring Chart
Circle what your heart decides to do

9 WEEK LIFE TRANSFORMATION
SCORING CHART

Name: _____

Date: from _____ to _____

WEEK	CHAPTER	ELEMENT	DATE	SCORE
1	2	Water		_____ /1
2	3	Greens		_____ /1
3	4	Sugar		_____ /1
4	5	Fat		_____ /1
5	6	Minerals		_____ /1
6	7	Exercise		_____ /1
7	8	Moon		_____ /1
8	9	Spirit		_____ /1
9	10 & 11	Metabolism & Heart		_____ /2

TOTAL POINTS: _____ /10

9-10 PTS: Consider yourself healthy!
6-8 PTS: You'd be healthier if you made serious changes
5 OR LESS: You need a complete lifestyle overhaul

FINAL THOUGHTS

This book was written to testify the **unlimited power of God's love.** God gave you all the power to heal yourself from all illnesses. With His almighty power, He designed and created you to heal from any disease. Because God is perfect and you are made in His image, you are perfectly designed. In other words, your body, mind, and spirit are whole, self sufficient, and self contained.

As you learned throughout this book, when you tinker with and taint what God created, your natural health turns to sickness and death. But when you use only God-given foods, drinks, air, thoughts, feelings, and beliefs, you will **find and maintain perfect health**. Be warned, however, that health can only be maintained by developing an intimate personal relationship with God. This requires you to just believe that you were created for the purpose of loving and communicating with your creator. When you have this belief in your heart, it will entrain all of your body to be perfectly healthy.

Once you attain health and wellness in your body, mind, and spirit, you are ready to carry out your mission and purpose in your life. This **personal mission** is from God. God made each and every one of us to fulfill our personal purpose of His creation. I hope and pray that this book has helped you to see the whole picture and that now, you are more equipped to take on the exciting journey of your life. May God be with every step of the way!

9WEEKTRANSFORMATION.COM
"CREATING WELLNESS EVANGELISTS"

Transformation means changing all three levels of being: body, mind, and spirit. The first level, transforming the body, means to metamorphose in form, appearance, or structure. This is the physical level of change. The second level, transforming the mind, is to convert in condition, nature, or character. The third level, transforming the spirit, means to transmute completely into another substance. Both the second and third levels of change are non-physical—they are mental and spiritual.

Truly transforming your mind, body, and spirit takes hard work, but it is possible, especially with guidance. My **9 Secrets Seminar Series** will give you the guidance you need to make important changes in your life. The transformation takes place over a series of empowering and inspiring educational seminars, which are meant to help participants makeover their lives in the areas of health, success, career, business, finance, and relationships.

THE SEMINARS

This site, **www.9WeekTransformation.com**, is the place that all my seminar participants will visit to search for information regarding upcoming programs, past seminars, and all the products I recommend. The site is designed to create **Wellness Evangelists,** people who have gone through the programs successfully and who are eager to testify and share their success stories with the rest of the world.

I believe wellness refers to getting healthy in every area of your life. That means developing healthy lifestyles, satisfying careers, successful businesses, stable finances, and happy relationships. All of these areas of life need to improve if you are to be truly well. Additionally, all people need to improve in the three levels of body, mind, and spirit. Most wellness programs available today only focus on one or two levels. I believe that is insufficient. A perfect balance of attention to body, mind, and spirit is the key to successful wellness programs. That's what you'll get with my 9 Week Transformation programs.

SEMINAR GOALS

The Web site and my seminar series both have two main goals, both of which are evident in the butterfly logo on the site. The first is called the **"incubation effect."** I once read a story about a man who saw a butterfly struggling to free itself from a cocoon on a window sill. Out of compassion, the man made a slit in the cocoon with a sharp knife, so the butterfly could get out. To his surprise, the butterfly could not fly away. The butterfly needed that time of struggle and incubation to gain strength to fly. In my seminars, the nine weeks make up that incubation period, which will get you ready to fly. Once you pass the struggle, you will be able to fly with vigor on your own, just as the logo shows.

The second goal of the site and series is appropriately called the **"butterfly effect."** One flap of a wing can create a typhoon on the other side of the world; in other words, what starts small can have a tremendous long-term effect. As seminar participants become **Wellness Evangelists**, their experiences will create a huge wellness force throughout the whole world.

WHAT YOU WILL ACCOMPLISH

When you participate in my seminar series, you will realize for the first time how God created the entire universe as a mirror image of everything that has life. This is the true meaning behind creation in His own image. You will learn that the Universal Law of God governs all aspects of your life, from your health and successes to your business ventures and relationships. After being empowered and inspired by this knowledge, you will understand all the unanswered **"why"** questions that you've wondered about before. Then, you will realize **"how"** life works and will know **"what"** to do to find your purpose. Unfortunately, most seminars start with **"what"** and never get to the most important things, the **"why"** questions. This is why you are not empowered by these programs. My seminars start with the most important information—the whys.

As the subtitle of this book says, **God truly gave you all the power to heal yourself.** Hopefully, after reading this book, you will understand that simple-yet-beautiful concept. We are in the worst economic, ethical, and moral turmoil of all time. It is time for us to get up and depend on ourselves. We need to be the drivers of our own destinies. We need to truly learn how to empower ourselves. This requires both the belief that we can heal and the practical knowledge of how to do it. The Web site and my seminar series will be that inspiration and empowerment. And they will also be the practical knowledge to show you how to heal.

One more important thing about the seminars: I call my seminar series **"Edutainment."** I don't want you to come to another boring seminar. My series will be educational and entertaining at the same time. When you are having fun, you will truly be open to metamorphose, convert and transmute into a new you! So please join me in this exciting journey to transform every aspect of who you are. The following seminars are available for you to participate in.

9 SECRETS SEMINAR SERIES "TRANSFORMING YOU"

⤳ 9 Week LIFE Transformation ⤳

9 Secrets of Health
"Unlocking All Your God Given Power to Heal"

9 Secrets of Healthy Feet
"Preventing Breakdown"

9 Secrets of Healthy Back
"Generating Power"

9 Secrets of Stress Reduction
"Letting Go"

9 Secrets of Healthy Daily Living
"Creating Great Habits"

9 Secrets of Salt
"Unlocking the Healing Power of Natural Salt"

∽ 9 Week SUCCESS Transformation ∽

9 Secrets of Success
"Unlocking Your Service Habits"

9 Secrets of Time Management
"Prioritizing"

9 Secrets of Leadership
"Magnetizing"

9 Secrets of Team
"Building Master Mind Alliances"

9 Secrets of Adversity Management
"Celebrating"

∽ 9 Week BUSINESS Transformation ∽

9 Secrets of Business of Life
"Unlocking Your Prosperity Mindset"

9 Secrets of Marketing
"Branding You"

9 Secrets of Management
"Systemizing"

9 Secrets of Money Management
"Disciplining"

⌇ 9 Week RELATIONSHIP Transformation ⌇

9 Secrets of Relationships
"Unlocking Your True Happiness"

9 Secrets of Family Relationships
"Accepting"

9 Secrets of Couples' Relationships
"Becoming One"

WELLNESSEVANGELISTS.ORG
"TESTIFYING THE GOOD NEWS OF WELLNESS"

When you participate and experience my 9 Secrets Seminar Series, you will undergo two different stages. During the seminar, you will be a partner to someone going through the same transformative process. After you've completed your nine weeks, you'll be a **mentor** who will encourage other people to get involved and transform their ways. If you choose to participate further, you can then become a **leader** at the seminar for a group of participants. If you would like to get even more involved, you can become a **facilitator** or a **speaker** for your community or a group. As soon as you start teaching others about transforming themselves on any level, you have become a **Wellness Evangelist**.

Wellness Evangelists (WE) are those who are transformed or are transforming every aspect of their lives to become new people. **WE** cannot help but talk about their transformation with everyone they meet. **WE** share and testify how faith has healed them from worldly misery and brought eternal love. **WE** testify how they have transformed their worldly lives to be more influential, more prosperous, and happier.

WellnessEvangelists.org is all about you. You that transformed or who is in the process of transforming. This is your site! This is the site where you can share and testify how you have healed from all your diseases, your unsuccessful life habits, your poverty-stricken mindset, and your unhappy relationships. This is the site to spread your good news of wellness to the rest of the world, so that others will be inspired to replicate your success. We want to hear that you overcame illnesses, you reconnected with God, you found your true purpose in life, you learned to serve more people, and you healed family separations. We want to hear about these and many more success stories.

If you have any transformational success stories as a **Wellness Evangelist, WellnessEvangelists.org** wants to hear from you. When you first visit **WellnessEvangelists.org**, you will be given a **WE** member number and a password. Please provide accurate personal information. Your personal information will only be used for **WE** usage and nothing else. **WE** want to protect you and your loved ones.

I so look forward to hearing your stories through our website and hopefully in person at one my seminars. I am extremely anxious for that time!

ACKNOWLEDGMENTS

Special thanks to all the wonderful teachers and authors who made the concepts and details of this book possible. Many authors I have read did not make it into the notes of this book, but they still taught me a great deal. The following notes list all the authors whom I quoted from.

NOTES

INTRODUCTION

1   Hendel, Barbara and Peter Ferreira. *Water and Salt: The Essence of Life*. Natural Resources Inc., 2003. 33.

2   "Heart Lessons." The Science Museum of Minnesota. <www.smm.org.>

3   "Heart Lessons."

4   "The Cardiovascular System." *Your Gross and Cool Body*. Discovery Channel Online. <www.yucky.discovery.com>

5   Xie, Min. *Fundamentals of Robotics: Linking Perception to Action*. Hackensack, NJ: World Scientific, 395.

6   Farndon, John. *The Human Body*. Orgeon City, OR: Marshall Cavendish, 4.

7   Farndon 4.

8   Farndon 4.

9   Campbell, Neil et al. *Biology*. Benjamin Cummings, 2007. 802.

10   Everett, Lesley. *Drop Dead Brilliant*. New York: McGraw-Hill, 2007. 32.

11   Medina, John J. *The Clock of Ages: Why We Age, How We Age, Winding Back the Clock* Cambridge UP, 1997. 93.

12   Murakami, Kazuo. *The Divine Code of Life*. Atria Books, 2006. 1-2.

13   Murakami 1-2.

14   Lipton, Bruce. *The Biology of Belief*. Hay House, 2008. 53.

15   Palladino, Michael. *Understanding the Human Genome Project*. San Francisco: Pearson, 2006. 7.

16   Church, Dawson. *The Genie in Your Genes*. Santa Rosa, Ca.: Energy Psychology Press, 2009. 35-36.

17   Lipton 34.

18   Ruby, Margaret. *The DNA of Healing*. Charlottesville, Va.: Hampton Roads Publishing Co., 2006.13.

19   Lipton 37.

20   Lipton 39

21   Lipton 42.

22   Church 37.

CHAPTER 1

23   Lesmoir-Gordon, Nigel et al. *Introducing Fractal*. Cambridge, UK: Totem Books, 2006. 3.

24   Lesmoir-Gordon et al. 7.

25   Lesmoir Gordon et al. 148.

26   Mandelbrot, Benoit. *The Fractal Geometry of Nature*. New York: W.H. Freeman and Co., 1983. 204-205.

27   Lesmoir-Gordon et al. 85.

28   Lesmoir-Gordon et al. 76.

29   Lesmoir-Gordon et al. 108-109.

30   Lesmoir-Gordon et al. 111.

31   Gerard, Robert V. *Change Your DNA, Change Your Life!*. Coarsegold, Ca.: Oughten House Foundations Inc., 2000. 9.

32   Lesmoir-Gordon et al. 134.

33   McEvoy, J.P. and Oscar Zarate. *Introducing Quantum Theory*. Cambridge, UK: Totem Books, 2007. 19.

34   McEvoy and Zarate 75.

35   Lipton 70-71.

36   Lipton 68-69.

37   Pagels, Heinz R. *The Cosmic Code*. New York: Bantam, 1984. 243.

38   Bloom, William. *The Endorphin Effect*. London: Platkus, 2001. 42.

39   Meade, Michael as qtd. in Masuro Emoto. *The Healing Power of Water*. New York: Atria Publishing, 2001. 215.

CHAPTER 2

40   Cousens, Gabriel and David Rainoshek. *There Is a Cure for Diabetes*. North Atlantic Books, 2008. 261.

41   Brody, Jane. *The New York Times's Guide to Personal Health*. New York: Times Books, 1982. 63

42   Moritz, Andreas. *Timeless Secrets of Health and Rejuvenation*. Enerchi.com, 2007. 30.

43   Alcamo, Edward and Jeffrey Pommerville. *Alcamo's Fundamentals of Microbiology*. Jones & Bartlett Publishers, 2006.55

44   Chaplin, Martin. "Information Exchange Within Intracellular Water." *Water and the Cell*. Eds. Gerald Pollock et al. Springer Books, 2006. 114.

45   Belen, Susana. *Detox and Revitalize: The Holistic Guide For Renewing Your Body, Mind, and Spirit*. Vital Health Publishing, 2005. 144.

46   Colbin, Annemarie. *Food and Healing*. New York: Ballantine Books, 1986. 220.

47   See the end of this chapter for more information.

48   Watson, Brenda and Leonard Smith. *The Detox Strategy*. Free Press, 2009. 141.

49   Connolly, M.A. *Communicable disease control in emergencies: a field manual*. World Health Organization, 2006. 295.

50   Vasey, Chris. *The Water Prescription*. Rochester, Vermont: Healing Arts Press, 2002. 10.

51   Holloway, William D. and Herb Joiner-Bey. *Water: Foundation of Youth, Health, and Beauty Water: Foundation of Youth, Health, and Beauty*. New York: IMPAKT Health, 2002. 6.

52   Vasey.

53   Batmanghelidj. *Your Body's Many Cries For Water*. Falls Church, Va.: Global Health Solutions, 1997. 115

54   Batmangheldj 115.

55   Batmangheldj 115.

56   Batmanghelidj. *Water Cures, Drugs Kill*. Falls Church, Va.: Global Health Solutions, 2003. 27.

57   Batmanghelidj, *Your Body's Many Cries for Water*. 41.

58   Batmangheldj 41.

59   Batmangheldj 48.

60 Vasey 149.

61 Parsons, Kenneth C. *Human Thermal Environments*. CRC, 2002. 69.

62 Cruise, Jorge. *The 3-Hour Diet*. Collins, 2006. 81.

63 Vasey. 12-13.

64 Vasey 12-13.

65 Duyff, Roberta Larson. *American Dietetic Association Complete Food and Nutrition Guide*. Wiley, 2006. 156.

66 Duyff 44.

67 Newman, Bettina et. al. *Lose Weight the Smart Low-Carb Way*. Rodale, 2002. 260.

68 Batmanghelidj, F. *Water for Health, for Healing, for Life*. New York: Warner Books, 2003.

69 Garrett, William E. and Donald Kirkendall. *Exercise and Sport Science*. Lipincott, Williams & Wilkins, 2000. 146.

70 Gillenwater, Jay Young et al. *Adult and Pediatric Urology*. Lipincott, Williams & Wilkins, 2002. 536.

71 Aj,Djo and Bill Quinn. *The Hot Diet*. Thomas Nelson, 2007. 55

72 Braun, Stephen. *Buzz*. New York: Oxford U P, 1996. 6.

73 Cherniske, Stephen. *Caffeine Blues*. New York: Warner Books, 1998. 63.

74 Cherniske 48-49.

75 Braun 108.

76 Cherniske 6.

77 Cherniske 27.

78 Weinberg, Bennett and Bonnie Bealer. The Caffeine Advantage. New York: The Free Press, 2002. 13.

79 Chernske 52.

80 Cherniske 51.

81 Cherniske 85.

82 Cherniske 322.

83 Cherniske 303.

84 Braun 6.

85 Braun 39, 68.

86 Braun 66.

87 Horner, Christine. *Waking the Warrior Goddess*. Basic Health Publications, 2007. 42.

88 Natow, Annette and Jo-Ann Heslin. *The Protein Counter*. New York: Pocket Books, 2003. 1.

CHAPTER 3

89   Lipton 53-56.

90   Lipton 32.

91   Boutenko, Victoria. *Greens For Life*. San Diego: Raw Family Publishing, 2005. 47

92   Wolfe, David. *The Sunfood Diet Success System*. San Diego: Maul Brothers, 2001. 232.

93   Boutenko 186.

94   Wolfe 81.

95   Eades, Michael and Mary Eades. *Protein Power*. New York: Bantam, 1996. 191.

96   Young, Robert O. and Shelley Redford Young. *The pH Miracle*. New York: Warner Books, 2002. 5.

97   Young and Young 28.

98   Young and Young 28.

99   Young and Young 28.

100   Young and Young 28.

101   Vasey, Christopher. *The Acid-Alkaline Diet*. Rochester, Vermont: Healing Arts Press, 1999. 17-19.

102   Prescott, David M. and Abraham Flexer. *Cancer: The Misguided Cell*. Sinauer Associates Inc, 1986. 30.

103   Miller, Edwin Cyrus. *Plant Physiology with Reference to the Green Plant*. McGraw-Hill, 1938. 545.

104   Wigmore, Ann. *The Sprouting Book*. Avery Trade Books, 1986. 12.

105   Wolfe 187.

106   All entries are taken from *The Protein Counter*.

107   Market, Dieter. *The Turbo-Protein Diet*. Houston: BioMed International, 2000. 78-79

108   Market 82.

109   Market 82.

110   Boutenko 53.

CHAPTER 4

111   Bennett and Sinatra. *Sugar Shock!* New York: Berkley Books, 2007. 37.

112   Bennett and Sinatra introduction.

113   Brand-Miller, Jennie et al. *The New Glucose Revolution*. New York: Marlowe & Co., 2003.11.

114   Fittante, Ann. *The Sugar Solution*. New York: Rodale, 2006. 3.

115   Bennett and Sinatra 37.

116   Woodruff, Sandra. *The Good Carb Cookbook*. New York: Avery, 2001. 6.

117   DesMaisons 24.

118   DesMaisons 25.

119   Appleton, Nancy. *Lick the Sugar Habit*. New York: Avery, 1996. 201.

120   Eades and Eades 193.

121   Oski, Frank. *Don't Drink Your Milk!* New York: Teach Services, 1993. 3.

122   Oski 10.

123   Oski 35.

124   Oski 50.

125   Bennett 143.

126   Brand-Miller et al. 23-24.

127   Brand-Miler et al 33.

128   Chart taken from Gallop, Rick. *The G.I. Diet*. New York: Workman Publishing, 2002. 10.

129   Woodruff 71.

130   Brand-Miller et al. 37.

131   Brand-Miller et al 37.

CHAPTER 5

132   Erasmus, Udo. *Fats that Heal, Fats the Kill*. Vancouver: Alive Books, 1993. 155.

133   Vigilante, Kevin and Mary Flynn. *Low-Fat Lies: High-Fat Frauds*. Washington, D.C: Lifeline Press, 1999. 26.

134   Simopoulos, Artemis P. *The Omega Diet*. New York: HarperCollins, 1999. 19.

135   Kowalski, Robert E. *The New 8-Week Cholesterol Cure*. New York: Quill Books, 2002. 10.

136   Erasmus 64-65.

137   Kowalski 10.

138   Hirsch, Anita. *Good Cholesterol, Bad Cholesterol*. New York: Marlowe & Co., 2003. 74.

139   Kowalski 27-29.

140   Castelli, William P. and Glen C. Griffin. *The New Good Fat Bad Fat*. Tucson: Fisher Books, 1997. 83.

141   Kowalski 33.

142   Cooper, Kenneth H. *Controlling Cholesterol the Natural Way*. New York: Bantam, 1999. 22.

143   Hirsch 22.

144   Cooper 22.

145   Allport, Susan. *The Queen of Fats*. Berkeley, Calif.: U of California P, 2006. 21.

146   Hirsch 20-21.

147   Castelli 17.

148   Castelli 22-23.

149   Erasmus 55-57.

150   Simopoulos 5.

151   Hirsch 15.

152   Simopoulos 59.

153   Simopolous 33.

154   Simopoulos 33.

155   Simopoulos 29.

156   Castelli 56.

157   Erasmus 62-63.

158   Erasmus 125.

159   Erasmus 125.

160   Sears, Barry. *Toxic Fat*. Nashville, Tenn.: Thomas Nelson, 2008. 51.

161   Sears 3.

162   Simopoulos 25.

CHAPTER 6

163   Wallach, Joel and Ma Lan. *Rare Earths Forbidden Cures*. Wellness Publications, 1994. 48

164   Wallach and La*n* 39.

165   Wallach and Lan 44.

166   Wallach and Lan 44.

167   Feinstein, Alice, ed. *Prevention's Healing With Vitamins*. New York: Rodale Books, 1998. 9

168   Colbert 181.

169   Feinstein 45.

170   Colbert 184.

171   Wallach, Joel and Ma Lan. *Dead Doctors Don't Lie*. Wellness Publications, 2004. 367.

172   Feinstein 53.

173   Feinstein 54-55.

174   Colbert 186-197; Feinstein 52.; Pederson, Mark. *Nutritional Herbology*. Whitman Publishers, 1998. 15.

175   Wallach and Lan. *Rare Earth*. 477.

176   As qtd. in Mindell, Earl and Hester Mundis. *Earl Mindell's New Vitamin Bible*. Grand Central Publishing, 2004. 5.

177   Wallach and Lan.. *Rare Earth*. 169.

178   Wallach and Lan. *Dead Doctors Don't Lie*. 226.

179   Wallach and Lan 84.

180   Mindell and Mundis 7.

181   *Nature's Plus: Natural Vitamin Handbook*. Natural Organics, 2004. 12-15.

182   Wallach and Lan. *Rare Earths*. 255.

183   Wallach and Lan 256.

184   Wallach and Lan 263.

185   *Nature's Plus*. 16-19.

186   Colbert 205.

187   Colbert 206-212.

188   Bauer, Brent, Ed. *Mayo Clinic Guide to Alternative Medicine 2007*. Time Inc, 2007. 19.

189   Bauer 19.

190   Colbert 200-204.

191   Mindell and Mundis 31.

192   Colbert 216.

193   Pederson 6.

194   Pederson 183.

195   Colbert 220.

196   Colbert 220.

197   Mindell and Mundis 11.

198   Weber, George. *Protecting Your Health With Probiotics*. IMPAKT Communications, 2001. 1.

199   Weber 19.

200   Weber 19.

201   Weber 20-21.

202   Starr, Joyce. *God's Guru on Natural Salt Wealth*. Aventura, Fla.: God's Guru Publishing, 2007. 16.

203   Brownstein, David. *Salt: Your Way to Health*. West Bloomfield, MI: Medical Alternatives Press, 2006. 17.

204   Starr 3.

205   Kulansky, Mark. *The Story of Salt*. New York: Putnam and Sons, 2006. 6.

206   Kulansky 7.

207   Kulansky 8.

208   Zronik, John Paul. *Salt, Rocks, Minerals and Resources*. New York: Crabtree Publishing, 2004. 16.

209   Strom, Laura. *The Rock We Eat*. New York: Children's Press, 2007. 8.

210   Strom 10, 24-25.

211   Kulansky 16.

212   Kulansky 39.

213   Strom 25.

214   Starr 84.

215   Kulansky 7.

216   Starr 28-29.

217   Brownstein 75.

218   Zronik 11.

219   Gutelius, Scott et al. *True Secrets of Salt Lake City Revealed.* Key West: Eden Entertainment, 2002. 45.

220   Starr 42.

221   Brownstein 26-27.

222   Brownstein 109.

223   Hendel and Ferreira 113.

224   Brownstein 30.

225   Brownstein 79-80.

226   Brownstein 60.

227   Brownstein 44-45.

228   Brownstein 46.

229   Brownstein 47.

230   Brownstein 118-119.

231   Brownstein 110-111.

232   Hendel and Ferreira 108.

233   Brownstein 68.

234   Hendel and Ferriera 180/

235   Starr 55.

236   Starr 56-57.

237   Hendel and Ferriera 184.

CHAPTER 7

238   Donovan, Sara. *Mall Walking Madness.* Rodale Books, 2006. 31.

239   Egoscue, Pete and Roger Gittiness. *The Egoscue Method of Health Through Motion.* New York: Quill Books, 2001. 47.

240   Egoscue 36.

241   Egoscue 64.

242   Egoscue 32, 37.

243   Chart information from Colbert 119-126.

244   Kortge, Carolyn Scott. *The Spirited Walker.* San Francisco: Harper Collins, 1998. 4.

245   Fife, Bruce. *The Detox Book: How To Detoxify Your Body To Improve Your Health.* Picadilly Books, 1997. 108.

246   Malkin, Mort. *Aerobic Walking: The Weight-Loss Exercise.* New York: John Wiley and Sons, 1995. 1.

247 Hahn, Frederick et al. *The Slow Burn Fitness Revolution: The Slow-Motion Exercise That Will Change Your Body In 30 Minutes A Week.* New York: Broadway Books, 2003. 20.
248 Hahn et al 21.
249 Egoscue 5.
250 Donovan 128.
251 Egoscue 15.
252 Kortege 172.
253 Malkin 1.
254 Donovan 32-33.
255 Rippe, James M. and Ann Ward. *The Rockport Walking Program.* New York: Prentice Hall Press, 1989. 17.
256 Malkin 157.
257 Kortge 178.
258 Kortge 3.
259 Kortge 22.
260 Isaacs 8.
261 Fenton, Mark and David R. Bassett Jr. *Pedometer Walking: Stepping Your Way to Health, Weight Loss, and Fitness.* Guilford, Conn.: The Lyons Press, 2006. 127.
262 Fenton and Bassett 76.
263 Kortge 9.
264 Kortge 9..
265 Fenton and Bassett 35.
266 Fenton and Bassett 35.
267 Fenton and Bassett 94.
268 Malkin 10.
269 Brittenham, Dean and Greg Brittenham. *Stronger Abs and Back.* Champaign, Ill.: Human Kinetics, 1997. Ix.
270 Brittenham and Brittenham 9.
271 Kortge 104.
272 Mittleman, Stu. *Slow Burn: Burn Fat Faster By Exercising Slower.* New York: Quill Books, 2000. 106.
273 Farhi, Donna. *The Breathing Book.* New York: Henry Holt and Co., 1996. 55.
274 Farhi 55.

CHAPTER 8

275 Lipton 97.
276 Murphy, Joseph. *The Power of Your Subconscious Mind.* Radford, Va.: Wilder Publications, 2007. 104.

277   Lipton 140.

278   Murphy 118.

279   Servan-Schreiber, David. *The Instinct To Heal: Curing Stress, Anxiety, and Depression Without Drugs.* New York: Rodale Books, 2004. 26.

280   Lipton 97

281   Lee, Ilchi. *Brain Wave Vibration.* Sedona, AZ: Best Life Media, 2008. 22.

282   Leyden-Rubenstein, Lori. *The Stress Management Handbook.* New Canaan, Conn.: Keats Publishing, 1998.10.

283   Childre, Doc and Deborah Rozman. *Transforming Stress.* Oakland, Ca.: New Harbinger Publications, 2005. 57-58.

284   Childre and Rozman 85.

285   Ready, Romilla and Kate Burton. *Neuro-Linguistic Programming for Dummies.* Chichester, England: John Wiley & Sons, 2004. 54.

286   Leyden-Rubenstein 68-69.

287   Lipton 117-118.

288   Colbert 229.

289   Childre and Rozman 85.

290   Campbell, Adam. "The Anatomy of a Potbelly." *Best Life.* Oct. 2006. 89.

291   Childre and Rozman. 86

292   Childre and Rozman 86.

293   Cecil, Russell LaFayette et al. *Cecil Textbook of Medicine.* 23rd Edition. Saunders, 2007. 1253.

294   Childre and Rozman 87.

295   Childre and Rozman 2.

296   Childre and Rozman 33.

297   Childre and Rozman. 34.

298   Leyden-Rubenstein 30.

299   Leyden-Rubenstein 56.

300   Lipton 132.

301   Lipton 132-133.

302   Leyden-Rubenstein 75.

303   Lipton 134.

304   Lipton 134.

305   Lee 35.

306   Leyden-Rubenstein 81-82.

307   Lee 22.

308   Lee 59.

309   Ready and Burton 57.

310   Yoo, JinSo. *Restoring the Image of God.* 15.

311   Kraft, Charles K. *Deep Wounds, Deep Healing*. Ventura, Ca.: Regal, 1993. 16.

312   Yoo 46-47.

313   Yoo 46-47.

314   Yoo 46-47.

315   Yoo 46-47.

316   Yoo 44.

317   Yoo 44.

318   Yoo 60.

319   Yoo 76.

320   Yoo 106

321   Foster, Russell G. and Leon Kreitzman. *Rhythm of Life*. New Haven: Yale UP, 2004. 249.

322   Smolensky, Michael and Lynne Lamberg. *The Body Clock Guide to Better Health*. New York: Henry Holt and Co., 2000.

323   Foster 144.

324   Epstein, Lawrence J. *A Good Night's Sleep*. New York: McGraw Hill, 2007. 22.

325   Foster and Krietzman 249.

326   Epstein 196.

327   Smolensky and Lamberg 109.

328   Murphy 86.

329   Epstein preface, 37-38.

330   Colbert 45.

331   Colbert 51.

332   Epstein 4-5.

333   Colbert 45.

334   Colbert 37.

335   Colbert 45.

336   Colbert 43-44.

337   Epstein 18.

338   Colbert 14.

339   Colbert 31

340   Colbert 8.

341   Colbert 55-65.

342   Colbert 88-90.

343   Smolensky and Lamberg 111.

344   Leyden-Rubenstein 156.

345   Epstein 20.

346   Colbert 57-60.

347   Leyden-Rubenstein 112.

348   Leyden-Rubenstein 113.
349   Leyden-Rubenstein 115.
350   Leyden-Rubenstein 118.
351   Leyden-Rubenstein 132.
352   Leyden-Rubenstein 134.
353   Leyden-Rubenstein 149.
354   Leyden-Rubenstein 159.

CHAPTER 9

355   Simon, Seymour. *Our Solar System.* 9.
356   Rau, Dana. *Earth.* 4.
357   Lydolph, Paul. *The climate of the earth.* 15.
358   Winrich, Ralph. *The Sun.* 4.
359   List take from Sears, Al and John Herring. *Your Best Health Under the Sun.* Wellington, Fla.: Al Sears, 2007. xviii-xix.
360   Sears and Herring 122.
361   Sears and Herring 162.
362   Sears and Herring 177-178.
363   Sears and Herring 184, 197.
364   Sears and Herring 219-220.
365   Sears and Herring 4.
366   Sears and Herring 201.
367   Sears and Herring 204.
368   Sears and Herring 38.
369   Sears and Herring 41.
370   Sears and Herring 47.
371   Sears and Herring 50.
372   Sears and Herring 53.
373   Sears and Herring 57-60.
374   Sears and Herring 63.
375   Sears and Herring 111.
376   Sears and Herring 208.
377   Sears and Herring 220.
378   Sears and Herring 230.
379   Sears and Herring 73.
380   Sears and Herring 73.
381   Sears and Herring 244.
382   Sears and Herring 244.
383   Sears and Herring 256.
384   Murphy 111.
385   1 Corinthians 13:4-7.

386   Mark 12: 28-31.
387   Chapman, Gary. *The Five Love Languages*. Chicago: Northfield Publishing, 2004.
388   Quiz from Chapman 199-202.
389   Bloom, William. *The Endorphin Effect*. London: Platkus, 2001. 83.
390   Bloom 74-76.
391   Bloom 97.
392   Bloom 102.
393   Bloom 127.
394   Prager, Dennis. *Happiness Is a Serious Problem*. New York: Regan Books, 1998. 15.
395   Prager 19.
396   Prager 27.
397   Prager 31.
398   Prager 101
399   Prager 150.
400   Prager 123.
401   Prager 146.
402   Prager 156.
403   Bloom 21.
404   Bloom 21.
405   Plotnikoff, N.P. et al. "Ying-Yang Hypothesis of Immunomodulation." *Enkephalins and Endorphins*. New York: Plenum Press, 1986. 1.
406   Bloom 6.
407   Bloom 7.
408   Bloom 26-27.
409   Heubner, Hans. *Endorphins, Eating Disorders, and Other Addictive Behaviors*. New York: W.W. Norton & Co., 1993. 17-18.
410   Heubner 29
411   Emoto, Masaru. *The Hidden Messages in Water*. New York: Atria Publishing, 2001. 5.
412   Weston, Walter. *How Prayer Heals*. Charlottesville, Va.: Hampton Roads Publishing Co., 1998. 7.
413   Weston 9.
414   Miller, Robert. *Miracles in the Making*. Atlanta: Ariel Press, 1996. 120.
415   Miller 116.
416   Miller 115.
417   Miller 48.
418   Miller 111-114.
419   Miller 195-196.

420   Proverbs 4:20-22.

421   Wimber, John and Kevin Springer. *Power Healing*. San Francisco: Harper Collins, 1991. 35.

422   Wimber and Springer 36.

423   Wimber and Springer 41.

424   Kuhlman, Kathryn. *A Glimpse of Glory*. South Plainfield, NJ: Bridge Publishing, 1983.3.

425   Kulman 57.

426   Wimber and Springer 66.

427   Wimber and Springer 80.

428   Wimber and Springer 100.

429   Wimber and Springer 157.

CHAPTER 10

430   David, Marc. *Mind/Body Nutrition*. Nightingale Conant, 2006. 3.

431   Schwarzbein, Diana. *The Program*. Deerfield Beach, Fla.: Health Communications Inc, 2004. 10.

432   David 7-8.

433   David 8.

434   David 9.

435   David 14-15.

436   Malkmus, George. *The Hallelujah Diet*. Destiny Image Publishers, 2006. 192.

437   Simontacchi, Carol. *The Crazy Makers*. London: Penguin, 2000. 102-106.

438   Blaylock, Russell. *Excitotoxins*. Santa Fe, NM: Health Press, 1997. 34.

439   Statham, Bill. *Eat Safe*. Philadelphia: Running Press, 2008. 22.

440   Roberts, H.J. *Aspartame, Is it Safe?* Philadelphia: Charles Press, 1990. 28.

441   Roberts 48.

442   Statham 61, 86.

443   Farlow, Christine. *Food Additives*. Escondido, Calif.: KISS for Health Publishing, 2007. 49, 62.

444   Statham 99.

445   Shaw, Judith. *Transfats*. New York: Pocket Books, 2004. 9.

446   Farlow 67.

447   Farlow 80.

448   Farlow 31.

449   Farlow 105-106.

450   Farlow 31.

451   Farlow 108.

452   Statham 163.

453   Farlow 108.

454   Farlow 22.

455   Hyman, Mark. *Five Forces of Wellness*. Nightingale Conant, 2006. 125.

456   Hyman 30.

457   Hyman 52.

458   Hyman 69.

459   Hyman 84.

CHAPTER 11

460   Childre and Martin. *The Heartmath Solution*. New York: HarperOne, 2000. 9.

461   Childre and Martin 38.

462   Childre, Doc and Bruce Cryer. *From Chaos to Coherence*. Boulder Creek, Ca.: Planetary, 2004. 13.

463   Childre and Martin 33.

464   Childre and Martin 30.

465   Childre and Martin 10.

466   Childre and Martin 30.

467   Childre and Martin 55.

468   Childre and Martin 35.

469   Childre and Martin 15.

470   Exercise taken from Childre and Martin 213-214.

471   Frankl, Viktor. *The Will to Meaning*. New York: Penguin, 1980. ix.

472   Frankl 34

473   Warren, Rick. *The Purpose Driven Life*. Grand Rapids, Mich.: Zondervan, 2002. 17.

474   Childre and Martin. 92.

475   Childre and Martin 98.

476   Table from Plasker, Eric. *The Longevity Solution*. Nightingale Conant, 2008. 11-12.

477   Evans, Dylan. *Placebo*. New York: Oxford UP, 2004. 2-3.

478   Thompson, Grant. *The Placebo Effect and Health*. Amherst, N.Y.: Prometheus Books, 2005. 17.

479   Thompson 21, 109.

480   Lipton 110.

481   Evans 80.

482   Kuby, Lolette. *Faith and the Placebo Effect*. Novato, Ca.: Origin Press, 2001. 67.

483   Kuby 32.

484   Thompson 15.

485   Thompson 152.

486   Kuby 68.

487   Evans 200.

488   Kuby 16.

489   Kuby 7, 13.

490   Kuby 232.

491   Kuby 238.

492   Lipton 111.

493   Thompson 15.

494   Lipton 112.

495   Thompson 279.

496   Hill, Napoleon. *Think and Grow Rich*. Radford, Va.: Wilder

       Publishing, 2007. 72.

ABOUT THE AUTHOR

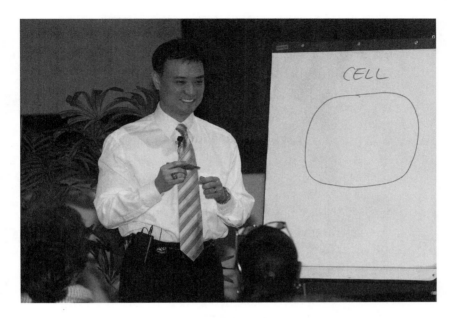

Dr. S. Don Kim is a board certified foot and ankle surgeon who specializes in reconstructive ankle surgeries. Since 1991, he has been the medical director of the Los Angeles based Kim Foot and Ankle Medical Centers.

Dr. Kim has been an innovator in the health, nutrition and fitness fields for more than a decade. He discovered that the human body, mind and spirit are the mirror images of the universe. Dr. Kim postulates that by understanding the qualities and patterns of the universe, we can better understand how our body, mind and spirit work together.

Dr. Kim is passionate about educating, empowering and inspiring all people. He hopes his lessons will enable success in the areas of health, business, career management, finance and personal relationships. Dr. Kim believes that empowering education is the key to a prosperous and balanced life. He has conducted hundreds of life-changing seminars since 2002.

PRODUCT INFORMATION

If you would like more information about
all of the organic products that were
mentioned in this book, please go to
www.**9WeekTransformation.com**
or www.**VitaManna.com**.

There, you will find information about:

· VITAMANNA® (MorningManna®, MiddayManna®,
EveningManna®) — a combination of vitamins,
minerals, antioxidants, digestive enzymes,
probiotics, and phytonutrients.
· SLEEPMANNA® – natural sleep aids.
· SALTMANNA® – encapsulated natural salt.
· GREEN, GREEN, GREENS® – organic green powder.

To purchase and receive more information about Dr. Kim's
books, please visit his website **www.9Secrets.com**.

If you would like more information about salt therapy and
salt products, please go to www.**9WeekTransformation.com**
or www.**SaltandtheLight.com**.

You may contact Dr. Kim directly at
Kim Foot and Ankle Medical Centers, Inc.
701 E. 28th Street Suite 111
Long Beach, CA 90806
(562) 426-2551

Or visit Dr. Kim's website www.**KimFoot.com**.